COPING
WITH
ARTHRITIS

by

**Othniel J. Seiden, MD
& Jane L. Bilett, PhD**

Cover Art
by Capri Brock

A Books To Believe In Publication
All Rights Reserved
Copyright 2009 by Othniel Seiden & Jane L. Bilett

Proudly Published in the USA by
Boomer Book Series

BoomerBookSeries.com

ISBN: 151941353X

DEDICATIONS

To Dr. David Wiener
& the Orthopedic Department of
Kaiser Permanente - for replacing
both of my arthritic hips...

TABLE OF CONTENTS

Appendices
Appendix I: Quit Smoking Now ™
Appendix II: Arthritis statistics

Recommended Reading

Other books by Seiden & Bilett

About the Authors

PREFACE
AND PURPOSE

This book ***Coping With Arthritis*** is written as a part of the Boomer Book Series **www.BoomerBookSeries.com** because of the huge number of Baby Boomers and senior citizens that are afflicted with one or another form of this disease. Furthermore, the number of arthritis patients is growing at a rapid rate. This is not to infer that arthritis is only a disease of the elderly, Arthritis in its varied forms affects children, teens and young adults in surprising numbers however it is more widely accepted as a process of aging.

An estimated 46 million adults in the United States reported having been told by their physicians or health advisors that they have some form of arthritis, rheumatoid arthritis, gout, lupus, or fibromyalgia. That's one in every five adults in the United States alone. By the year 2030, it is estimated that over 67 million of Americans aged 18 years or older will have medically diagnosed arthritis of one form or another. A surprising statistic to most people is that almost 300,000 children under age 18 have one or another form of arthritis, representing approximately one in every 250 children.

The most common form of arthritis is osteoarthritis.

An estimated 21 million adults have osteoarthritis. Other prevalent related conditions include gout, fibromyalgia and rheumatoid arthritis. Another estimated 2.1 million adults suffer from rheumatoid arthritis. Gout has been diagnosed in an estimated 5.1 million adults and it is estimated 3.7 million more adults have fibromyalgia. These figures have been generated by the National Center for Disease Control.

It is the purpose of this book to give these patients and their families a clear understanding of the many and varied diseases that fall under the heading of **Arthritis.** We will focus on prevention measures and treatments available for each.

CHAPTER 1

WHAT IS ARTHRITIS?
DEFINITION AND OVERVIEW

Arthritis is inflammation of one or more of your joints usually resulting in pain, swelling, stiffness, and limitation of motion. Arthritis includes over 100 different types of joint diseases.

The most common of these are osteoarthritis and rheumatoid arthritis. Arthritis is the breakdown of cartilage that normally protects the joints, allowing them smooth movement. Cartilage is also a shock absorber when pressure or sudden impact is placed on the joints, as when you jog, jump, walk or lift heavy weight. Without a healthy amount of cartilage at the joints, the bones may rub together, causing pain, inflammation, swelling, heat pain and stiffness.

Joint pain and inflammation may be due to a variety of reasons, including broken bones, healed fractures and other injuries. Bacteria or viruses, an Autoimmune disease (meaning the body attacks itself because the immune system mistakenly reacts to a body part as if it were a foreign object), can cause general wear and tear on joints causing joint pain. Usually in some of these, the inflammation goes away after the injury heals or the disease is cured or the infection clears.

However, with some injuries and diseases, the inflammation does not go away or destruction causes long-term or chronic pain and deformity known as chronic arthritis.

Of all forms of arthritis, osteoarthritis arthritis is the most common type and the most likely to affect the general population.

Osteoarthritis may affect any joint, but most commonly, it will occur in the hips, knees, ankles, feet or fingers.

Risk factors for osteoarthritis include, being overweight, previously injuring an affected joint, using the affected joint in a repetitive action putting excessive stress on the involved joints.

Other types or causes of arthritis include:
* Rheumatoid arthritis in adults
  Juvenile rheumatoid arthritis in children
* Systemic lupus erythematosis or SLE
* Gout
* Scleroderma
* Psoriatic arthritis
* Ankylosing spondylitis
* Reiter's syndrome or reactive arthritis
* Adult Still's disease
* Viral arthritis
* Gonococcal arthritis
* Other bacterial infectious arthritics

❖ Fibromyalgia
❖ Tertiary Lyme disease
❖ Tuberculosis arthritis
❖ Blastomycosis or other fungal infectious arthritis

Arthritis in all its forms ranks the number one most common causes of disability in the United States.

Common as arthritis in all its forms is, there still abound many myths about it so let us dispel some of the more common ones.

Myth: Only older people get arthritis.
In fact: Older people do get arthritis, but so do children. However, two-thirds of all arthritis patients are younger than 65, some of the most serious forms of arthritis occurring in teenagers and people under thirty. Arthritis is a chronic disease and people live with this forever.

Myth: There is not much anyone can do to combat arthritis.
In fact: There are many things that can be done, including physical therapy, pool exercise, medications, and as a last resort, surgery and joint replacement. Some arthritis responds to diet and weight reduction.

Myth: Cracking your knuckles causes arthritis.
In fact: It just isn't so. There is absolutely no evidence that suggests that cracking one's knuckles can cause arthritis.

Myth: Exercise flares arthritis symptoms.

In fact: It is just not true, actually, the most important thing society can do is to encourage people to exercise and walk. Exercise and activity helps build muscle strength and maintain stability of affected joints. Activity slows the progression of arthritis and keeps one limber. Inactivity increases stiffness and pain.

Myth: Once arthritis strikes, it's a downhill slide to total disability.

In fact: In just the last decade, there have been so many advances in our understanding of arthritis, its causes and treatment, that people should be very optimistic about their future.

Symptoms

If you have arthritis, some of the symptoms you may experience might include:

❖ Joint pain
❖ Joint swelling
❖ Joint stiffness especially in the morning or after inactivity
❖ Warmth or heat around the affected joint
❖ Redness around the affected joint
❖ Difficulty moving the joint through its full range of motion

Diagnostic signs and tests

Your doctor will first want to take a detailed medical history to differentiate if arthritis or some other musculoskeletal problem might be the cause for your symptoms. Next, he or she will carry out a thorough physical examination. An examination of the affected joints may show that fluid, called an "effusion," has collected around the joints. The joint may be tender to touch or when gently pressed, and may be warm and red. Each joint will be put through a range of motion to measure its function and limitation. It may be uncomfortable or difficult to rotate indicating a limited range of motion. In some forms of arthritis or autoimmune diseases, the joints may become deformed if the disease is untreated. These are often signs of severe, untreated rheumatoid arthritis.

Following a complete history and examination your physician will more than likely order laboratory tests. These tests will vary depending on the suspected types of arthritis. They probably include blood tests, perhaps examination of joint fluid and probably joint x-rays. To check for infection and other causes of arthritis like gout joint fluid is simply and painlessly removed from the joint with a needle and examined under a microscope or by cultures to diagnose the specific types of arthritis.

Treatments
Treatments of arthritis vary with the specific types of arthritis and the joints affected, the severity or the disease and how it affects your daily activities. Age and occupation will also be taken into consideration when the doctor creates a specific treatment plan for you. Treatment will first focus on eliminating the underlying cause of the arthritis whenever possible. However, the cause may not be curable, as in the case of osteoarthritis or rheumatoid arthritis. In addition to cure of cause where possible, focus will be to reducing your pain and discomfort, gain you maximum return of function and prevention of further disability.

It may be possible to treat the problem by just making some lifestyle changes and without medications.

If needed, medications should be used in moderation and in addition to lifestyle changes. Lifestyle changes may be aimed at weight reduction, diet quality and reduction of trauma to the joints. Exercise for arthritis is necessary to maintain healthy joints, relieve stiffness, reduce pain and fatigue, and improve muscle and bone strength. All exercise programs should be tailored to the individual. It is likely a physical therapist or personal trainer will work to design an individualized program. It will probably include range of motion exercises to improve flexibility, strength training for muscle tone and low-impact aerobic activity to improve endurance. Pool exercises and swimming may also prove beneficial. Physical therapists may also apply heat and cold treatments as needed and fit the patient for splints or orthotics, devices to support and align joints. This may be particularly necessary for rheumatoid arthritis. Physical therapists may also consider water therapy, ice massage, or transcutaneous nerve stimulation also known as TENS.

Rest is as important as exercise. Sleeping 8 to 10 hours per night and taking naps during the day may aid the recovery from a flare-up. Rest may be instrumental in helping prevent exacerbations. In addition, the patient should avoid positions or movements that place extra stress on the affected joints. Avoid inactivity and holding one position for long periods of time. Reducing stress, (which can aggravate symptoms) is another key element to quick recovery. The physical therapist may endorse the use of yoga and tai chi.

Alternative medical treatments such as acupuncture, massage, or chiropractic may be recommended and helpful. Occupational therapists may be called upon to help you modify your home to make activities easier and safer like having grab bars in the shower, the tub, near the toilet and moving objects that could trip you or cause falls.

Other treatment measures may include taking Glucosamine and/or Chondroitin that are thought to be building blocks of cartilage. These are supplements available over the counter and may reduce osteoarthritis symptoms. Alteration of your diet making it rich in vitamins and minerals, especially antioxidants found in fruits and vegetables may be helpful.

MEDICATIONS

Your doctor will choose from a variety of medications as needed. The first drugs he or she may recommend may be available without a prescription. These include Acetaminophen or Tylenol and Aspirin, Ibuprofen or Naproxen. If more varied medications are needed your physician will turn to prescription medicines. These will vary greatly with the type of arthritis you have and will be discussed in greater detail when covering treatments for the individual varieties of the disease.

SURGICAL AND OTHER APPROACHES

In some cases, surgery to rebuild the affected joint may be necessary. This is called arthroplasty. In some cases, it may require actual replacement of the affected joint to achieve and maintain a more normal lifestyle. The decision to perform surgery is generally made after other alternatives have been exhausted and are no longer effective. Healthy joints contain synovial fluid that lubricates the joint. In arthritic joints, this fluid may not be adequately produced. Your doctor may suggest injecting the arthritic joint with a manmade version of joint fluid. This synthetic fluid may postpone the need for surgery at least temporarily and improve the quality of life for persons with arthritis. This injection may also include cortisone and a local anesthetic. Such an injection may give relief of symptoms for up to several months.

A few anatomic and physiologic definitions

Cartilage is a layer of tissue at the end of bones making up a joint that cushion joints against impact and allows freedom of smooth motion. It is gel-like, porous, and elastic when healthy.

Articular surface is the area inside the joint where the ends of the bones meet.

Bone remodeling is a process in which a damaged bone attempts to repair itself. .

Collagen is the main protein found in bone tendon, cartilage, skin, and connective tissue.

Osteophytes are outgrowths, spurs or lumps developed at the joint end of bones. They usually develop due to excessive pressure on the joint.

Synovium is the membrane found lining the inner surface of joints that secretes a fluid that lubricates the joint to avoid friction.

Subchondral bone refers to that part of a bone under the cartilage.

CHAPTER 2

OSTEOARTHRITIS OVERVIEW

Osteoarthritis is a chronic condition caused by the breakdown of the affected joint's cartilage. Cartilage is the cushion part of the joint at the ends of the bones that allows easy movement of joints. The breakdown of this cartilage allows the bones to rub against each other, resulting in stiffness, pain and loss in range of movement. Osteoarthritis has come to be known by many names, which include degenerative joint disease, osteoarthritis, hypertrophic arthritis and degenerative arthritis.

Evidence of osteoarthritis has been found in earliest humans and ice-aged skeletons. **Today, almost 30 million Americans live with osteoarthritis, also abbreviated as OA.** Causes of OA include age, obesity, injury or overuse and genetics. Frequently, it is brought about by a combination of any of these potential causes.

Osteoarthritis develops in stages. At first, cartilage loses elasticity as we age and thus is more easily damaged by injury or use. This wear and damage of cartilage causes changes to underlying bone. Increased friction and stress on the bone causes thickening at the joint end and cysts may occur under the protective cartilage. Often bony growths, called spurs or osteophytes, develop at the affected joint. Bits of bone or cartilage may break away and float loosely in the joint space. These loose particles, (often called joint mice), further damage the remaining cartilage. The joint lining, (or the synovium), becomes inflamed and causes inflammatory proteins called cytokines and other enzymes to form in the joint that further damage and break down cartilage. All of these changes in the joint cartilage and bones eventually lead to pain, stiffness and limitation of movement and mobility.

In time, this deterioration of cartilage can affect the shape and makeup of the joint so it will not function normally and smoothly. Joint mice floating freely in joint fluid causes irritation and pain and sometimes seem to 'lock up' the joint. Bony spurs, or osteophytes, when they develop only add to discomfort and diminished function. As joint fluid production is reduced by the damaged and aging cartilage, the joint's ability to absorb shock is diminished. With time, as severity increases osteoarthritis involves the entire joint and surrounding tissues including the nearby muscles, underlying bone, ligaments, joint lining, and the joint covering known as the joint capsule.

Diet & Osteoarthritis

It is quite widely accepted that diet strongly influences the development of osteoarthritis, either as a direct cause or as a contributory factor to other causes.

There is no question that obesity or excessive weight increases the risk for developing osteoarthritis. Obesity is a direct end to excessive food ingestion. Overweight people reduce their chances for developing or aggravating their osteoarthritis by losing weight. Losing weight also improves the chances of rehabilitating a joint already suffering osteoarthritis.

Vitamin C is essential to the development of normal cartilage. A deficiency of vitamin C might lead to the development of weak cartilage and onset of osteoarthritis. Vitamin C is found in citrus fruits and supplementation with vitamin C tablets may be advised if dietary fruits are unavailable.

People with low bone mineral density, such as in osteoporosis, may be at increased risk for osteoarthritis. Exercise and adequate calcium and vitamin D intake, as recommended for age and gender, can help to maintain bone density. Vitamin D deficiency increases the risk of joint space narrowing and progression of osteoarthritis. Some physicians recommend vitamin D supplementation of 400 IU daily.

For some years now, there have been studies suggesting that the food supplements Glucosamine and/or Chondroitin can help to relieve osteoarthritis symptoms. There is no strong evidence that Glucosamine alone, or in combination with Chondroitin, is of any real value in rebuilding cartilage that has been damaged by osteoarthritis.

Signs and symptoms

The main symptom of osteoarthritis is chronic pain, causing the loss of mobility and stiffness. The pain of osteoarthritis is usually described as a sharp piercing ache, or a burning sensation in the associated muscles, tendons and joints. OA can cause "crepitus" or a crackling noise in the affected joint when it is moved or touched. Patients may also experience muscle spasm and painful contractions in the affected tendons. The arthritic joints may also swell with excess fluid. OA most commonly affects the hands, feet, spine, and the large weight bearing joints like the hips, knees, ankles and feet. However, any joint in the body may potentially be affected.

In smaller joints, like in wrists, hands and fingers, hard bony enlargements, called Heberden's nodes might form on the distal interphalangeal or finger joints and/or Bouchard's nodes found on the proximal finger joints. They may not necessarily be painful, but they do significantly limit the movement of the fingers. OA of the toes leads to the formation of bunions, rendering them painful, red and swollen. Osteoarthritis is also the most common cause of *"water on the knee,"* which is an accumulation of excessive fluid in or around the knee joint. This is usually the result of trauma or excessive and chronic irritation of the joint.

Causes

Although OA is most commonly brought on from trauma, osteoarthritis very often affects multiple members of the same family, suggesting a hereditary susceptibility to this disease. There is a prevalence of the disease between siblings and especially among identical twins, indicating a genetic connection. Up to 60% of OA cases seem to have a genetic relationship. Studies also indicate the possibility of allergies, infections and fungi as causes. To help simplify and categorize osteoarthritis by its causes, it can be divided into primary and secondary arthritis.

Primary arthritis

Primary arthritis is a degenerative disorder related to aging. As a person ages, the liquid content of the cartilage decreases causing the cartilage to become less resilient. Without the protective effects of the proteoglycans which make up this liquid the collagen fibers of the cartilage become more susceptible to degeneration and damage. Inflammation can occur in the joint and surrounding tissues as breakdown products from the cartilage are released into the joint space. With time, the inflammation and irritation causes new osteophytes to form on the margins of the joints. In time, these bony changes and the increased inflammation they themselves cause can become extremely painful and debilitating.

Secondary arthritis

This type of osteoarthritis is caused by other predisposing factors or diseases which initiate the onset of arthritis. The final resulting osteoarthritis is the same as for primary OA. Predisposing causes of secondary osteoarthritis include genetic or congenital disorders such as abnormally formed joints, inflammatory diseases, gout, trauma and injury to joints, infections involving joints, sports injuries and even pregnancy, among other factors.

Diagnosis of osteoarthritis

The diagnosis of osteoarthritis is usually done through x-ray. X-rays will readily show the loss of cartilage, bone cysts, the narrowing of the joint space between the articulating bones, forming osteophytes. Other techniques, such as magnetic resonance imaging or MRI, arthroscopy and arthrocentesis may also be employed when x-rays are inconclusive. Laboratory tests may also be utilized but often these are to determine cause or to differentiate osteoarthritis from other similar diseases.

Treatment of osteoarthritis

The treatment of osteoarthritis is aimed at preventing further development of the disease and easing its symptoms to restore as much function and normal lifestyle for the patient.

For the most part, osteoarthritis is an irreversible disease and the best hope of treatment is to arrest its progression. Typically treatment consists of anti-inflammatory medication or other interventions that can reduce the pain of OA thereby improving the function of the involved joints. Physical therapy and exercise programs will help restore flexibility, strength and function to a degree.

Conservative care should always be tried before prescription medications and invasive or surgical treatment is utilized. Among early conservative treatments the most common is Chiropractic care. It is aimed at reducing incorrect joint alignments in hopes of preventing future progression and degeneration of the arthritic joints. Weight reduction and control, adequate rest and well designed exercise and mechanical support devices are all useful conservative forms of therapy.

Medical treatment

After all conservative efforts have been exhausted treatment with medications may be initiated. Medical treatment may begin with over the counter anti-inflammatories and pain reducers such as aspirin, ibuprofen, acetaminophen and naproxen. Following these over the counter meds, physicians may turn to stronger prescription drugs including the Non-steroidal meds or NSAIDs. In addition, cortisone and local anaesthetics may be use, often actually injected into the joints.

Acetaminophen
Acetaminophen is a mild pain reliever. The most popularly recognized brand is Tylenol. Its pain relief may be adequate in early and mild cases of osteoarthritis. Avoid taking it in large doses as it can be very liver toxic in overdose. Acetaminophen does not treat the inflammation of OA.

Non-steroidal anti-inflammatory drugs
Non-steroidal anti-inflammatory drugs NSAID may be used in more severe cases to reduce both the pain and inflammation. These include aspirin, ibuprofen and naproxen. High doses are often required. All NSAIDs act by inhibiting the formation of prostaglandins, which play a central role in inflammation and pain. These drugs may cause stomach upset, cramping, diarrhea, and peptic ulcer.

COX-2 selective inhibitors
These are another type of NSAID. COX-2 selective inhibitors have a better track record for the reduction of

inflammation, pain and progression of OA, but they have an added risk for cardiovascular disease and some have had to be withdrawn from the market.

Corticosteroids

Many doctors now avoid the use of steroids as their effect is modest and the adverse effects may outweigh the benefits. When used, it is usually only for short periods for acute flare-ups and often as injections.

Narcotics

For more to severe pain, narcotic pain relievers such as opiates such as hydrocodone, oxycodone or morphine may be indicated. Addiction is a danger if used for lengthy periods.

Topical and injections

There are a myriad of topical treatments for pain of arthritis of all types. These are treatments designed for local application. Some NSAIDs are available as topicals and may improve symptoms without having their systemic side-effects. Such creams and lotions may be effective in treating pain and inflammation associated with OA if applied with sufficient frequency.

Severe pain in specific joints may be treated with local lydocaine injections or other local anesthetic often in conjunction with corticosteroids. This is often "half time treatment" of athletic injuries such as sprains and stretch joint injuries. It places the joint in great jeopardy of further and permanent injury

In recent years, many dietary supplements have been tried in the treatment of osteoarthritis.

Glucosamine
A molecule derived from glucosamine is utilized by the body in renewing cartilage and synovial fluid. Supplemental glucosamine may improve the symptoms of OA and delay its progression. To date, studies have not unquestionably proven this. Never-the-less a great number of people use this over the counter product and will swear by it. There is no evidence indicating any risk to its use.

Chondroitin
Chondroitin sulphate, like glucosamine has become a widely used dietary supplement for treatment and prevention of osteoarthritis. It is frequently used in combination with glucosamine and studies have not proven it effective whether used alone or in combination. Its use also appears not to have any health risks.

Omega-3 fatty acid
Omega-3 fatty acid is a healthy fat supplement derived from deep water fish and has many health benefits especially for the heart and circulatory system. It is also widely used by osteoarthritis patients but its benefits are not certain.

Bromelain
This is an enzyme and thought by some to prevent and reduce inflammation. Its effectiveness is questionable.

Antioxidants
Many antioxidants, especially vitamins C and E as found in both foods and supplements, seem to provide pain relief from OA.

Hydrolyzed collagen

This supplement may also prove beneficial in the relief of osteoarthritis pain and limitation of motion symptoms. In a six month placebo-controlled German study of 100 elderly patients, the hydrolyzed collagen group showed significant improvement in joint mobility.

Ginger

Ginger extract has been found to moderately improve knee symptoms.

Selenium

Selenium's deficiency seems to correlate with a higher severity and progression of OA

Folate, vitamins B9 and B12

These vitamins when taken in large doses have been thought to reduce OA. There may be some down side risks in taking these vitamins in excessive doses.

Vitamin D

Vitamin D deficiency has been reported in OA patients and supplementation with Vitamin D is recommended for pain relief. It may also retard the progression of the disease.

Surgery

As a last resort, surgery and joint replacement may be indicated which have a very high success rate and can restore near normal function. If the above treatments and management are eventually ineffective, joint replacement surgery may be required. Individuals with very painful osteoarthritis joints may require surgery such as fragment removal, repositioning bones, fusing bone to increase stability and reduce pain and joint replacement.

Othniel Seiden, the author has had three hip replacement surgeries and will tell anyone his personal experience. Immediately after surgery, he felt better and had less pain than he'd experienced in over a year before the surgery. Recovery from hip surgery is quite easy as long as you follow through with physical therapy and exercise.

Of all joint replacements, hips are perhaps the easiest to endure, though in the past few years, knee surgeries have been much improved. Most joints are replaceable and can help return you to an active lifestyle. Age need not be a factor. When all else has been tried, do not hesitate getting a couple of surgical opinions and keep your options open.

Positive self-talk

As important as medications and other treatments are important to managing your pain and disability.

However another often overlooked yet major component to treatment is your attitude.

Attitude in the face of pain and disability often can determine what impact osteoarthritis will have on everyday lifestyle. Utilize positive self-talk. Self-talk is the endless stream of thoughts that run through your head day in and day out. These thoughts can be positive or negative. Too often self-talk arises from myth and misconceptions that were created from rumor or lack of information. Hopefully self-talk comes from logic and reason.

Most thoughts running through most people's heads are primarily negative. If that is the case, then the outlook on life is likely to be negative and pessimistic. If positive thoughts dominate, then likely optimistic thoughts will also, and that will lead to better coping with osteoarthritis or any illness or disease. It's important to keep a positive attitude.

Along with your doctor and family, make a plan for managing your arthritis. Knowledge that you're in charge of your disease, rather than your disease dictating to you will help you to cope. There is overwhelming evidence that people who take control of their treatment and with their doctors and an active support system, manage their arthritis better. They experience less pain and function far better. Above all, know your limits. Rest when you're tired. All forms of arthritis can fatigue you and cause muscle weakness. Frequent rest or short naps that do not interfere with nighttime sleep are very helpful.

If depression or frustration appear to be taking over, talk to your doctor. He or she may have ideas about how to better cope or even refer you to someone who can help.

CHAPTER 3

RHEUMATOID ARTHRITIS

Rheumatoid arthritis affects about two-million Americans in all ages and lifestyles. It is more prominent among women.

The disease is three times more common in women as in men. It afflicts people of all races equally.

The disease can begin at any age, but most often starts after age 40 and before 60. Multiple members in some families may be affected, suggesting a genetic basis for the disorder. This form of arthritis causes joint deformity marked by inflammation, stiffness, heat, redness, soft tissue swelling around the joints, pain and dysfunction. Rheumatoid arthritis is known to be an autoimmune disease that causing chronic inflammation of the affected joints and inflammation of the tissue around those joints. Furthermore, rheumatoid arthritis may affect other organs in the body as well.

Autoimmune diseases are a classification of illnesses that occur when the body tissues are mistakenly attacked by its own immune system. The immune system is a complex organization of cells and antibodies intended to seek out and destroy foreign invaders to the body, such as infections, pollens (in the case of allergies) and other pollutants dangerous to health.

Patients who have autoimmune diseases have antibodies in their blood that mistakenly target their own body tissues. Since rheumatoid arthritis (or RA) can affect multiple other organs of the body, it is often referred to as a systemic disease, sometimes called rheumatoid disease.

Rheumatoid arthritis is a chronic illness, one lasting for years. The good new is that patients may experience long periods of time symptom free. However, rheumatoid arthritis is usually a progressive illness that potentially causes permanent joint destruction and limitation of function.

Causes of rheumatoid arthritis

The basic cause of rheumatoid arthritis is still unknown even though it is a very active area of worldwide research. Infectious agents such as viruses, bacteria, fungi and allergens have been suspected but none has been proven as the cause. Some researchers believe that rheumatoid arthritis may be genetically inherited. Environmental factors also seem to play a causative role in rheumatoid arthritis. Recently, scientists have reported that smoking and tobacco use may increases the risk of developing rheumatoid arthritis. Whatever the exact trigger, the result is an immune system attacking one's own tissues, causing inflammation in the joints and occasionally other tissues of its own body.

Symptoms of rheumatoid arthritis

The symptoms of rheumatoid arthritis,

unlike osteoarthritis, may come and go, depending on changes in the degree of specific tissue inflammation.

Rheumatoid arthritis can be active when tissues are inflamed, or at times in remission, when tissue inflammation subsides. There is no predicting remissions, which can occur spontaneously or with treatment. Remissions may last for weeks, months, or even years. During the remissions, symptoms of the disease disappear, and patients generally feel quite well and normal. When the disease relapses and becomes active again the symptoms return. This return of the disease activity and its symptoms is referred to as a flare. Periods of flares and remissions are typical.

Active rheumatoid arthritis symptoms include fatigue, loss of appetite, low-grade fever, muscle and joint aches, and stiffness. It is during active flares that joints become red, swollen, painful, and tender. This occurs because the lining tissue of the joint becomes inflamed and produces excessive joint fluid or synovial fluid. Muscle or joint stiffness is usually most notable in the morning upon waking and after periods of inactivity. Rheumatoid arthritis commonly flares during other illness in the body.

Rheumatoid arthritis usually presents with multiple joints inflamed simultaneously and in a symmetrical pattern, both sides of the body being affected. Most often the small joints of both the hands and wrists are involved making simple daily tasks such as turning doorknobs and opening jars difficult. The small joints of the feet may also commonly involved making walking painful and often putting shoes on difficult. Rarely only one joint may be inflamed mimicking joint inflammation caused by other forms of arthritis, such as gout or joint infections. Chronic inflammation may cause systemic damage to body tissues, cartilage and bone possibly resulting in joint deformity, destruction, and loss of function. Rheumatoid arthritis can even affect the cricoarytenoid joint that is responsible for the tightening of our vocal cords and change the tone of our voice, however this is a rare event. When this joint does become inflamed, it may cause hoarseness. Also, since rheumatoid arthritis is a systemic disease, it can cause inflammation of organs and areas of the body other than the joints, even the glands of the eyes and mouth causing dryness of these areas referred to as Sjogren's syndrome.

Rheumatoid inflammation of the lung lining called pleurisies causes chest pain with deep breathing or coughing. The lung tissue itself can also become inflamed, and sometimes nodules known as rheumatoid nodules develop within the lungs. Inflammation of the pericardium, the tissue surrounding the heart, called pericarditis, can cause a chest pain that typically changes in intensity when lying down or leaning forward. The rheumatoid disease can also reduce the number of red blood cells, or anemia, as well as the white blood cells making one more susceptible to infections. This decrease in white cells may be associated with an enlarged spleen referred to as Felty's syndrome.

Firm lumps under the skin called rheumatoid nodules may occur around the elbows and fingers. Usually these nodules do not cause symptoms, but occasionally they can become infected. Vasculitis is a rare but serious complication of long-standing rheumatoid disease. This is blood-vessel inflammation and can impair blood supply to tissues possibly leading to tissue death. This is most often presents as tiny black areas around the nail beds or as leg ulcers.

Diagnosing rheumatoid arthritis

The diagnosis of rheumatoid arthritis should be made by a qualified physician because it can easily be mistaken for other similar diseases. Your doctor will review the history of symptoms, examines the joints for inflammation and deformity, the skin for rheumatoid nodules, and other parts of the body for inflammation. He or she will want to order certain blood and x-ray tests. The diagnosis will be based on the pattern of symptoms, the distribution of the inflamed joints, and the blood and x-ray findings. This may require several visits before your physician can be certain of the diagnosis. Your primary physician may refer you to another doctor with special training in arthritis and related diseases called a rheumatologist.

The distribution of joints inflamed is important to making a diagnosis.

In rheumatoid arthritis, the small joints of the hands, wrists, feet, and knees are more typically inflamed, affecting both sides of the body in a similar pattern.

If only one or two joints are inflamed, the diagnosis becomes more difficult and the doctor may have to perform other tests to exclude arthritis due to infection, gout or other cause. The detection of rheumatoid nodules around the elbows and fingers, can suggest the diagnosis.

Laboratory testing can be very helpful in making a definitive diagnosis. There are abnormal blood antibodies found in 80% of patients with rheumatoid arthritis called rheumatoid factor. A blood antibody called Citrulline antibody, or also know as anti-citrulline antibody, anti-cyclic citrullinated peptide antibody, and anti-CCP, is present in most patients with rheumatoid arthritis. Citrulline antibodies have been found in the earlier stages of rheumatoid arthritis.

A third antibody called the antinuclear antibody or ANA is also frequently found in patients with rheumatoid arthritis. A less specific blood test called the sedimentation rate measures of how fast red blood cells settle to the bottom of a test tube. The sedimentation or sed-rate is usually faster during disease flares and slower during remissions. Another blood test used to measure the degree of inflammation present in the body is the C-reactive protein; however, the rheumatoid factor, ANA, sed-rate, and C-reactive protein tests can be abnormal in other systemic autoimmune and inflammatory conditions so they are not specific for RA. Consideration of all symptoms, history and blood tests have to be well thought-out and then x-rays will most likely be added to the diagnostic package.

Joint x-rays may actually be normal or only show swelling of soft tissues during early stages in the disease however as the disease progresses x-rays can show bony erosions in the joints typical of rheumatoid arthritis. Joint x-rays can also be very helpful in monitoring the progression of disease and joint damage over time. In addition, bone scanning, which is a radioactive test procedure, can identify inflamed joints.

Arthrocentesis

Your physician may want to perform an office procedure called arthrocentesis in which a sterile needle is used to drain joint fluid out of the joint for laboratory analysis. Its main value is to help to exclude other causes of arthritis, such as infection or gout. Arthrocentesis can also be used in relieving joint swelling and pain. Occasionally, cortisone medications and anesthetics may be injected into the joint through arthrocentesis in order to relieve joint inflammation and reduce painful and limiting symptoms.

Treatment of rheumatoid arthritis

As with osteoarthritis, there is no known cure for rheumatoid arthritis though it is prone to having periodic remissions.

Until further research progress is made, the goal of treatment for rheumatoid arthritis is to reduce joint inflammation and pain, maximize joint function, and prevent joint destruction and deformity.

Early medical intervention has been shown to be important in improving long-term outcome. Aggressive management pays in improved function, slowing damage to joints as seen on x-rays, and reducing loss of function and work disability. Optimally treatment for the disease control involves medications, rest, joint-strengthening exercises, joint protection, as well as patient and family education. Treatment should be customized to each patient according to his or her disease activity, joints involved, general health, age, and patient occupation and lifestyle.

Commonly two classes of medications are used in treating rheumatoid arthritis. These are classified as fast-acting (or first-line drugs) and slow-acting (or second-line drugs). Slow acting drugs are referred to as DMARDs, which stands for disease-modifying anti-rheumatic drugs.

The first-line drugs, such as aspirin, ibuprofen, naproxen, and corticosteroids, are used to reduce pain and inflammation. Acetylsalicylate (Aspirin), naproxen (Naprosyn), ibuprofen (Advil, Medipren, Motrin), and etodolac (Lodine) are examples of NSAIDs or non-steroidal anti-inflammatory drugs. NSAIDs are medications specific for reduction of tissue inflammation, pain, and swelling. NSAIDs are not cortisone hence the name "non-steroidal." Some side effects of aspirin and other NSAIDs include stomach upset, abdominal pain, sometimes ulcers and even gastrointestinal bleeding. In order to reduce these side effects, NSAIDs are usually taken with food or medications including antacids and proton-pump inhibitors.

Corticosteroid medications can be given orally or injected directly into tissues, joints, and are more potent than NSAIDs in reducing inflammation and in restoring joint mobility and function. Corticosteroids are best used for short periods during severe flares of disease activity or when the disease does not adequately respond to NSAIDs. Corticosteroids, if misused, can have serious side effects including weight gain, facial puffiness, thinning of the skin and bone, easy bruising, cataracts, increased risk of infection, muscle wasting, and destruction of large joints, such as the hips and also some increased risk of contracting infections.

The slow-acting second-line drugs on the, such as gold, methotrexate and hydroxychloroquine other hand promote disease remission and prevent progressive joint destruction. The second-line drugs are not anti-inflammatory agents. In some patients with severe joint deformity or debilitating pain and limitation, surgery may be indicated and considered.

Second-line slow-acting disease-modifying anti-rheumatic or DMARDS drugs

Rheumatoid arthritis control requires medications other than pain and anti-inflammatory NSAIDs and corticosteroids to stop progressive damage to cartilage, bone, and adjacent soft tissues. The medications needed for more complete management of the disease are referred to as disease-modifying anti-rheumatic drugs or DMARDs. These second-line or slow-acting medicines may take weeks to become effective. When effective, DMARDs can promote remission and retarding of progression of joint destruction and deformity. Second-line medications may be used together in combination therapy.

The various DMARD meds available include Hydroxychloroquine or Plaquenil a relation to quinine, which is used in the treatment of malaria. It is used over a long period in treatment of rheumatoid arthritis. Its possible side effects include upset stomach, skin rashes, muscle weakness, and visual changes; though vision changes are rare, patients taking Plaquenil should be monitored by an ophthalmologist.

Sulfasalazine (trade named Azulfidine) is an oral medication long used in the treatment of mild to moderately severe inflammatory bowel diseases, such as ulcerative colitis and Crohn's disease. Azulfidine is usually used in combination with anti-inflammatory medications used in the treatment of rheumatoid arthritis. Uncommon side effects include rash and upset stomach. It should be avoided by patients with known sulfa allergies.

Methotrexate has gained popularity as a second-line drug because of its effectiveness and infrequent side effects. Methotrexate an immune-suppression drug can affect the bone marrow and the liver but rarely causing cirrhosis. Regular blood test monitoring of blood counts and liver function should be required by all patients taking methotrexate require.

Gold salts have been utilized in the treatment of rheumatoid arthritis for most of the past century. Gold salts are given by injection, initially on a weekly basis for months to years. Oral gold was not made available until the 1980s. Side effects of gold include skin rash, mouth sores, kidney damage with leakage of protein in the urine, and bone marrow damage causing anemia and low white-cell count. Blood and urine tests monitoring is a must. Oral gold may also cause diarrhea.

D-penicillamine or Depen and Cuprimine are sometimes used in selected patients with progressive forms of rheumatoid arthritis. Side effects are similar to those of gold and include fever, chills, mouth sores, a metallic taste in the mouth, skin rash, kidney and bone marrow damage, stomach upset, and easy bruising. Patients on this medication also require routine blood and urine tests.

Immunosuppressive medicines are powerful drugs that suppress the body's immune system and a number of these are used to treat rheumatoid arthritis. They include methotrexate described above, azathioprine or Imuran, cyclophosphamide or Cytoxan, chlorambucil or Leukeran and cyclosporine or Sandimmune. Because of potentially serious side effects, immunosuppressive medicines are usually used for patients with very aggressive disease.

Newest treatments of RA

Newer "second-line" drugs for the treatment of rheumatoid arthritis include leflunomide or Arava and biologic medications that include etanercept or Enbrel, infliximab or Remicade, anakinra or Kineret, adalimumab or Humira, rituximab or Rituxan and abatacept or Orencia. In comparison with traditional DMARDs, the biologic medications have a much more rapid onset of action and can have powerful effects on stopping progressive joint damage. Leflunomide (Arava) is available to relieve the symptoms and halt the progression of the disease. It seems to work by blocking the action of an important enzyme that has a role in immune activation. Arava can cause liver disease, diarrhea, hair loss, and/or rash in some patients. It should not be taken just before or during pregnancy because of possible birth defects.

Additional treatments of benefit for RA

Regular exercise is important for maintaining joint mobility and in strengthening the muscles around the affected joints. Swimming is particularly helpful because it allows exercise with minimal weight bearing and stress on the joints. Physical and occupational therapy by trained therapists provide specific exercise instructions, can offer splinting, and supports for deformed and weakened joints; wrist and finger splints can be helpful in reducing inflammation and maintaining joint alignment. Heat and cold applications can ease symptoms of RA. Many devices, such as canes, toilet seat raisers, and jar grippers can assist daily living.

Surgery may be recommended to repair damaged joints and restore joint mobility. Types of joint surgery range from arthroscopy to partial and complete replacement of affected joint. Arthroscopy is a surgical technique where a physician inserts a tube-like instrument into the joint to see and repair abnormal tissues. Total joint replacements are surgical procedures where destroyed joints are replaced with artificial materials. Most common in RA are replacements of the small joints of the hand replaced with plastic joints and the large joints of the hips or knees replaced with metals and ceramics.

Psychologically, the minimizing of emotional stress can help improve the overall health of patients with rheumatoid arthritis. Support groups may benefit patients allowing them to discuss their problems with others and learn more about their illness.

A summary of RA

Rheumatoid arthritis is an autoimmune disease that causes chronic inflammation of the joints and other parts and organs of the body. It usually has remissions and flares. It can affect persons of all ages, women more often than males. The basic cause of rheumatoid arthritis is not known. Multiple joints are usually, but not always, affected in a symmetrical pattern often involving the small joints of the hands, wrists and feet. Chronic inflammation of rheumatoid arthritis can cause permanent joint destruction and deformity and aggressive treatment may minimize the amount of permanent damage caused. Rheumatoid factor is an antibody blood test that may be found in 80% of patients with the disease.

There is no known cure for rheumatoid arthritis aggressive treatment can hold symptoms and permanent damage to a minimum. Treatment of rheumatoid arthritis optimally involves combinations of patient education, rest, prudent exercise, joint protection, medications, and occasionally surgery. Early treatment of rheumatoid arthritis will usually result in better outcomes.

OTHER FORMS OF ARTHRITIS AND SIMILAR DISEASES

CHAPTER 4

GOUT

Sufferers of Gout, often called metabolic arthritis, are in pretty good company. Throughout history this disease has affected some quite famous names like Queen Anne of Great Britain, King George IV, King Henry VIII, Christopher Columbus, Benjamin Disraeli, Benjamin Franklin, Alexander Hamilton, John Hancock, Thomas Jefferson, Kublai Khan, Joseph Conrad, Alfred Lord Tennyson, Charles Darwin, Isaac Newton, Karl Marx, Nostradamus, John Calvin and Pope Clement VIII.

Gout is a disease caused by a buildup of uric acid in the blood and then cristalizing in the joints. Monosodium urate or uric acid crystals are deposited on the articular cartilage of various joints, tendons and surrounding tissues because of this elevated concentrations of uric acid in the blood stream. These crystals then provokes an inflammatory reaction of these tissues which is extremely painful.

Signs and symptoms of gout

Gout is usually characterized by sudden, excruciating, unexpected, pain, as well as swelling, redness, heat, and stiffness in the affected joint. A low-grade fever may also be present with flares of this diesase. Gout occurs most commonly in men, usually having its onset in the toes, but less often it can appear in other parts of the body and affecting women as well.

The crystals formed inside the joint cause intense pain whenever the area is moved and the inflammation of the tissues around the joint also causes the skin to be swollen, tender and sore if even slightly touched; even a sheet or blanket in contact with the affected area can cause extreme pain.

Gout usually attacks the distal joints of the feet when it first appears most often the big toe in 75% of all first attacks. As in everything there are always exceptions and in about 25%, gout may affect other joints early on, such as the ankle, heel, instep, knee, wrist, elbow, fingers, and spine. Patients with longstanding gout or hyperuricemia can develop uric acid crystal deposits called *tophi* in other tissues even to be felt in the outer ear and elevated levels of uric acid in the urine can lead to uric acid kidney and bladder stones.

Diagnosis

A definitive diagnosis of gout is easily made by light microscopy of a sample of fluid aspirated from the affected joints. Blood tests commonly performed are full blood count, electrolytes, renal function, thyroid function tests and erythrocyte sedimentation rate or ESR. This helps to exclude other causes of arthritis, most notably septic arthritis, and to find any underlying cause for the hyperuricaemia. Purine metabolism causes a rise to uric acid, which is normally excreted in the urine. When metabolism causes excessive uric acid in the blood or when uric acid is not adequately excreted by the kidneys, crystals are more likely to form. Purines may be generated by the body by the breakdown of cells in normal cellular turnover, or may be ingested in purine-rich foods such as seafood, meats and some vegetables. The kidneys are responsible for approximately two-third of uric acid excretion, with the intestines responsible for the rest. Defects in the kidneys may be genetically determined to be responsible for the predisposition of to develop gout. To further indicate a genetic basis for gout, there are different racial potentials for developing this disease. In the United States, gout is twice as prevalent among African American males as it is in European-Americans.

It is interesting that a significantly higher incidence of acute gout attacks occurring in the spring of the year. Gout affects mostly men between the ages of 50 to 60.

The high levels of uric acid in the blood are often caused by protein rich foods. Alcohol intake may also causes acute attacks of gout and hereditary factors may contribute to the elevation of uric acid. It has been noted that, persons with gout are usually obese, predisposed to diabetes and hypertension, and at higher risk of heart disease. Gout is more common in affluent societies due to diets rich in proteins, fat, and alcohol, however it may come as a consequence of other health conditions especially renal failure.

Treatment

For acute attacks, the first line of treatment should be aimed at pain relief. The drugs of choice for symptom relief are indomethacin, ibuprofen or other nonsteroidal anti-inflammatory drugs or NSAIDs, oral glucocorticoids, or intra-articular glucocorticoids administered via a joint injection. Colchicine was for a long time the drug of choice in acute attacks of gout usually relieving the pain within 48 hours. NSAIDs are now the preferred form of analgesia for patients with gout, although side effects like gastrointestinal upset, diarrhea and nausea can accompany, they have a faster onset. If taken with food or antacids these side effects can be minimized. NSAIDs such as ibuprofen can provide relief from inflammation and pain; NSAIDS such as aspirin should <u>never</u> be used as it can worsen the condition because it raises plasma uric acid levels even at low doses by inhibiting uric acid secretion by the kidneys.

The use of ice packs gives relief of pain and keeping well hydrated and heating the affected joint in hot water will promote the dissolving and clearance of the urate crystal deposits in the joints. Perhaps the best relief is to alternate cold and warm packs to affected joints. Keeping the affected area elevated above the level of the heart is usually quite helpful. For long-term management of gout professional medical care is strongly recommended. For *extreme* cases of gout it may be necessary to remove large tophi and correct joint deformity by surgery.

It is interesting that gout may be related to sleep apnea. This may be because insufficient oxygen to the body cells releases purines as a by-product of the breakdown of oxygen-starved cells. Treatment of apnea with a C-Pap machine can be effective in lessening incidence of acute gout attacks. If you are snoring excessively or suffer fitful sleep it would be wise to have a sleep study done.

Diet

Flesh foods such as beef and seafood are high sources of purine and greatly increases the risk of developing gout. Dairy products such as milk and cheese seem to significantly reduce the chances of gout.

Coffee consumption seems associated with a lower risk of gout. Unless uric acid levels are caused by other health conditions a diet low in purines reduces the serum level of uric acid.

All sources of dietary protein supply purines. Meat especially dark meat and seafood are high in purine because muscle cells are a major source of purines, so high consumption of meat and seafood were found associated with an elevated risk of gout flares. Men who drink two or more sugary soft drinks a day have an 85% higher risk of gout because soft drinks contain large quantities of high-fructose corn syrup which results in Hyperuricemia in blood. Consumption of beer has been associated with a 50% increase in increased risk, while consumption of stronger spirits was associated with only about a 15% increase in relative risk of gout flares and no association has been found with consumption of wine.

Food high in purines best to avoid include meat, fish, poultry, sweetbreads, kidneys, liver, brains, or other organ meats - seafood particularly shellfish such as clam, oyster, scallop, shrimp, crab, lobster, and crayfish, sardines and anchovies. Vegetables such as asparagus, cauliflower, mushrooms and spinach should be avoided during flares.

Fruit preserves, jam, jelly syrups and candy all high in sugars should be avoided at all times.

It is wise to drink plenty of liquids, especially water, to dilute and assist excretion of urates and to avoid diuretic foods or medicines

To emphasize the importance of diet in the flaring of gout, for years I spent some of my vacation time as a ship's doctor for Holland American Cruise Lines. I almost always had gout patients come to me on about the second or third day of a cruise with flares of their disease. One of the big perks of a cruise is the food, around the clock food ... very rich food and drink. If breakfast, lunch, afternoon snacks, seven course dinner and then a midnight desert or pizza buffet isn't enough you can order room service 24-7. By day two or three, passengers predisposed to gout came to visit the ship's clinic.

CHAPTER 5

LUPUS, DISCOID AND SYSTEMIC LUPUS ERYTHEMATOSIS OR SLE

Lupus is an autoimmune disease that may affect various parts of the body, including skin, joints, heart, lungs, blood, kidneys, brain, and nervous system. The body's immune system normally makes proteins called antibodies to protect us against viruses, bacteria, and other foreign materials invading our bodies. These invading foreign materials are called antigens. In the autoimmune disorder lupus, the immune system cannot tell the difference between its own body tissue cells and foreign substances. Thus, the errant immune system makes antibodies directed against itself. These mistaken antibodies are called autoantibodies and cause inflammation, pain and damage in various parts of the body. This inflammation is considered the primary feature of lupus and is characterized by pain, heat, redness, swelling and loss of organ and tissue function.

Fortunately, for most people, lupus is a mild disease

affecting only a few organs. However, for others, it may cause serious, possibly life-threatening physical problems. Less than 20,000 Americans develop lupus each year and according to the Lupus Foundation of America about 1.5 to 2 million or more Americans has one form or another of lupus. Over 90% of all people with lupus are women and occurring most often in women in their childbearing years between the ages of 15 and 45. Lupus is also more common in African Americans, Latinos, Asians, and Native Americans than in Caucasians here in the United States. **Some famous patients include Louisa May Alcott**, American author. **Michael Jackson**, pop superstar and **Ferdinand Marcos**, former Philippine president.

Classification

Lupus, as mentioned above, is a chronic autoimmune disease. Clinically, it can affect multiple organ systems which may include the heart, skin, joints, kidneys, and nervous system. Discoid lupus erythematosus is a skin disorder causing a red, raised rash on the face and scalp. Discoid lupus occasionally, but less often than 1 to 5% of all cases, develops into systemic lupus erythimitosis or SLE. There are several other types of lupus; but when the word lupus is used alone it refers to systemic lupus erythematosus.

Systemic lupus erythematosus is a chronic disease and can at times turn fatal; however this is far less often true because with recent medical advances, fatalities are becoming quite rare. In cases of SLE, the immune system attacks various body's cells, systems and tissue, resulting in inflammation and tissue damage. SLE may affect any part of the body, but most often attacks the heart, joints, skin, lungs, blood vessels, liver, kidneys, and nervous system.

The course of the disease is unpredictable, with periods of illness or flares alternating with remissions. Lupus is now treatable symptomatically, mainly with corticosteroids and immunosuppressants, but there is currently no actual cure for the disease, however the survival rates in patients with SLE in the United States, Canada, and Europe is approximately 95% at 5 years, 90% at 10 years, and 78% at 20 years disease duration.

Other sub-groups of SLE include:

- ❖ Drug-induced Lupus erythematosus which occurs equally in either sex
- ❖ Lupus nephritis, which is an inflammation of the kidneys caused by SLE,
- ❖ Subacute cutaneous lupus erythematosus, which causes nonscarring skin lesions on patches of skin exposed to sunlight
- ❖ Neonatal lupus, a rare disease affecting babies born to women with SLE.

Signs and symptoms

Diagnosis of Systemic Lupus Erathematosis can be quite elusive, with patients sometimes suffering unexplained symptoms for years. The most common initial and chronic complaints are fever, malaise, joint pains, myalgias, fatigue and at times possible temporary reduction or loss of cognitive abilities. Because these vague and transient symptoms and signs are so often seen in other diseases, they tend to delay the correct diagnosis of SLE. The more common first signs may be dermatological manifestations. About 30% of patients present with some skin problems and 65% will eventually suffer such symptoms at some point in their disease with 30% to 50% suffering from the classic *butterfly rash* associated with the

SLE. When patients first present as discoid lupus this will appear as a thick, red and scaly patches on the skin and often alopecia or hair loss and/or mouth, nasal, and vaginal ulcers

Patients will most often first seek medical attention for joint aches and pains usually involving the small joints of the hand and wrist, although all joints are at risk. The Lupus Foundation of America estimates that well over 90% of SLE patients will experience muscular or joint pain and inflammation at some time during the course of their illness. However lupus arthritis is less disabling and usually does not cause severe or permanent destruction of the joints. Fewer than 10% of people with lupus arthritis will develop deformities of the hands and feet or hip and knee joints.

Hematological manifestations such as anemia and iron deficiency may develop in as many as 50% of SLE patients, as well as low platelet and white blood cell counts. More complicating to an accurate early diagnosis of SLE is that some patients may present with inflammation of various parts of the heart, such as pericarditis, myocarditis, and endocarditis involving either the mitral valve or the tricuspid valve. Atherosclerosis or inflammation of blood vessels also tends to occur more often advancing more rapidly in SLE patients than in the general population.

Pulmonary and respiratory manifestations include inflammation of the lung and pleura causing pleuritis, pleural effusion, lupus pneumonitis, chronic diffuse interstitial lung disease, pulmonary hypertension, pulmonary emboli, pulmonary haemorrhage and shrinking lung capacity.

Renal involvement may present with painless blood in the urine or the loss of protein in the urine called proteinuria. Eventually, acute or chronic renal impairment may develop with lupus nephritis, leading to acute or end stage renal failure. Fortunately, because of early recognition and management end stage renal failure occurs in less than 5% of patients.

Neurological manifestations occur in about 10% of patients and may present with seizures or psychosis. One-third may show a positive test for abnormalities in the cerebrospinal fluid. Other rarer manifestations of SLE are Lupus gastroenteritis, lupus pancreatitis, lupus cystitis, autoimmune inner ear disease, parasympathetic dysfunction, retinal vasculitis, and systemic vasculitis.

Research indicates that SLE may have a genetic link since lupus does often run in families. This genetic factor seems to be triggered by environmental factors. These environmental triggers may trigger the initial onset as well as exacerbate existing lupus conditions. They may include certain medications such as antidepressants and antibiotics, extreme stress, exposure to sunlight, hormones, and infections. UV radiation has been shown to trigger the photosensitive lupus rash. Some research has implicated silicone gel-filled breast implants in producing antibodies to their own collagen tissues.

Drug reactions may induce drug-induced lupus erythematosus. This however is a reversible condition that usually occurs in treatment of long-term illness. Drug-induced lupus mimics systemic lupus, but symptoms generally disappear once a patient is taken off the medication that triggered the episode.

The American College of Rheumatology (ACR) has established eleven criteria to help diagnose patients as having SLE Patient should present with four of the below eleven symptoms simultaneously or serially.

1. Pleuritis which is inflammation of the membrane around the lungs or pericarditis which is inflammation of the membrane around the heart
2. Oral ulcers or nasopharyngeal ulcers.
3. Arthritis which may be nonerosive arthritis of two or more peripheral joints, with tenderness, swelling, or effusion.
4. Photosensitivity where exposure to ultraviolet light causes rash;
5. Blood findings of a hemolytic anemia a low red blood cell count or leukopenia white blood cell count, in the absence of drug; sensitivity
6. Renal disorders.
7. Antinuclear antibody test showing positive;
8. Immunologic disorders and/or false positive serological test for syphilis.
9. Neurologic disorders such as seizures or psychosis.
10. Malar or butterfly rash on the cheeks.
11. Discoid rash, red scaly patches on skin causing scarring.

Treatment

There is no known cure for SLE, so treatment is aimed at dealing with the symptoms which involves preventing flares and reducing their intensity and duration when they do occur. Means of preventing and dealing with flares, including drugs, exercise, alternative medicine, and lifestyle changes.

Drug therapy is variable because of the great variety of symptoms and organ system involvement among lupus patients. Mild or remittent disease may in some cases be safely left untreated. If treatment is required or advised nonsteroidal anti-inflammatory drugs and antimalarials may be used. When more intense flares occur, they may be treated with corticosteroids.

Disease-modifying antirheumatic drugs or DMARDs are sometimes used preventively to hopefully reduce the incidence of flares and lower the need for steroid use. DMARDs in common use are some antimalarials and immunosuppressants such as methotrexate and azathioprine. In very severe cases, medications that suppress the immune system such as corticosteroids and immunosuppressants may be used to control the disease. Patients who take steroids may develop unwanted side effects such as obesity, diabetes, and osteoporosis, puffy face, an unusually large appetite, and sleep disorders. Avoiding direct sunlight with sun-protective clothing and using strong sun block lotion can also be effective in preventing photosensitivity problems.

Advances in treatment in past decades have improved survival to the point where many patients can live relatively asymptomatically. The most common cause of death when it does occur is infection due to treatments for immunosuppression and resulting from medications used to manage the disease. After age 60, the disease tends to run a more benign course.

CHAPTER 6

SCLERODERMA

Scleroderma affects approximately 300,000 people in the United States alone and is about four times as common in women as in men. Juvenile scleroderma affects approximately 7000 children in the United States. Scleroderma is an autoimmune disease of the body's connective tissue being attacked by its own immune system. Scleroderma is characterized by the formation of scar tissue or fibrosis in the skin and organs of the body. This leads to thickening and hardening of involved areas giving a waxy appearance to the skin. Scleroderma, when it is widespread over and through the body, is referred to as systemic sclerosis.

The cause of scleroderma is not fully known, but Research has found evidence that genetics is an important factor; however, the environment appears also to play a vital role. These factors trigger an activation of the immune system, initiating injury to tissues that result in a reaction similar to scar tissue formation. The genes seem to cause a predisposition to developing scleroderma meaning that inheritance plays a partial role. It is not at all unusual to find other forms of autoimmune diseases in families of scleroderma patients. The disease, while frequently disabling, tends not to be fatal. The systemic type or systemic sclerosis can be fatal as a result of heart, kidney, lung or intestinal involvement and damage.

Signs and symptoms of scleroderma

The most evident symptom of scleroderma is usually a marked hardening of the skin and associated scarring. The skin may appear tight, waxy, reddish or scaly and the blood vessels may appear more visible. In some affected areas fat and muscle wastage may affect appearance and weaken the patient. Important factors to consider are the level of internal organ involvement and the total area involved in the disease. In general, the more skin that is involved, the more severe the case of scleroderma will be.

In the systemic form of the disease over 80% of the patients have vascular symptoms referred to as Raynaud's phenomenon or disease. During an attack, there is discoloration of the hands and feet especially in response to cold. Raynaud's disease normally affects the fingers and toes. The systemic form of scleroderma and Raynaud's may cause painful ulcers on the fingers or toes known as digital ulcers.

Involvement of other organs

Diffuse systemic scleroderma may cause musculoskeletal, pulmonary, gastrointestinal, renal and nervous system complications.

Musculoskeletal system

The first joint problems noticed by patients with scleroderma are typically non specific joint pains, eventually leading to arthritis, and discomfort in tendons and/or muscles. Joint mobility, especially of the small joints of the hand, may become restricted by skin thickening and scarring. Patients may also develop considerable muscle weakness and fatigue.

Lung symptoms

Impairment in lung function is almost universally seen by pulmonary function testing in patients with diffuse scleroderma; however, it does not necessarily cause shortness of breath or other symptoms. Some patients can develop pulmonary hypertension which is typically progressive, and lead to right sided heart failure. Other pulmonary complications in more advanced disease include aspiration pneumonia, pulmonary hemorrhage and pneumothorax.

Gastrointestinal symptoms

Systemic scleroderma can affect any part of the gastrointestinal tract, but the most common manifestation in the esophagus as reflux esophagitis, which may be complicated by benign narrowing of the esophagus. This is usually initially treated with acid suppression or antacids. Scleroderma may decrease motility anywhere in the gastrointestinal tract and the most common site of decreased motility is the esophagus and the lower esophageal sphincter, often leading to dysphagia and chest pain. As Scleroderma progresses, esophageal involvement from abnormalities in decreased motility may worsen due to progressive scarring. The small intestine may also become involved, leading to bacterial overgrowth and malabsorption of bile salts, fats, carbohydrates, proteins, and vitamins. The colon when involved may cause pseudo-obstruction or ischemic colitis. Patients having more severe gastrointestinal involvement may often become profoundly malnourished.

Kidney symptoms

The most serious clinical complication of scleroderma involves the kidney which may lead to a scleroderma renal crisis. Symptoms of scleroderma renal crisis are malignant hypertension, hyperreninemia, azotemia (or kidney failure) with accumulation of waste products in the blood and microangiopathic hemolytic anemia the destruction of red blood cells. Apart from the high blood pressure, hematuria or blood in the urine and proteinuria or protein loss in the urine may be first indicative signs of the problem.

Diagnosis

The American College of Rheumatology agreed upon diagnostic criteria for scleroderma and divided it into three types.

Diffuse scleroderma or progressive systemic sclerosis is the most severe form having a rapid onset, involving widespread skin hardening, will generally cause much internal organ damage, specifically in the lungs and gastrointestinal tract, and is generally more life threatening.

Limited scleroderma or Crest syndrome is far milder having a slow onset and progression. "CREST" is an acronym for the five main features: **Calcinosis, Raynaud's syndrome, Esophageal** dysmotility, **Sclerodactyly** and **Telangiectasia.** Skin hardening is usually confined to the hands and face while internal organ involvement is less severe. A much better prognosis is expected. Raynaud's phenomenon may precede scleroderma by several years in typical cases of limited scleroderma. Raynaud's phenomenon is due to vasoconstriction of the small particularly the hands and feet. It is classically characterised by a color change, first white, and then blue in the cold. Finally, red on rewarming.

The scleroderma may be limited to the fingers, known as sclerodactyly and usually spares the lungs and kidneys.

Morphea or linear scleroderma scleroderma is the third type and only involves isolated patches of hardened skin and there generally is no internal organ involvement.

Treatment

There is no cure for scleroderma, though there are treatments for some of the symptoms, including drugs that soften the skin and reduce inflammation. Topical treatment for the skin changes of scleroderma do not really alter the disease course, but may reduce or improve pain and ulceration. NSAIDs (or nonsteroidal anti-inflammatory drugs) can be used to ease painful symptoms. Steroids such as prednisone have limited benefit. Raynaud's phenomenon sometimes responds to nifedipine or other calcium channel blockers. The skin tightness may be eased systemically with methotrexate and cyclosporin.

Other treatments are dictated by the organ systems that are involved by systemic scleroderma.

CHAPTER 7

PSORIATIC ARTHRITIS

Psoriatic arthritis is an inflammatory condition affecting the joints of children as well as adults with psoriasis, a skin condition causing patches of thick, red inflamed skin to form on certain areas of the body. However, not everyone with psoriasis develops psoriatic arthritis, yet everyone with psoriatic arthritis has psoriasis. Most patients develop the skin signs of psoriasis first. Best estimates indicate that about 10% to 15% of people with psoriasis will eventually develop psoriatic arthritis. Psoriasis is a skin condition affecting about 2% of the Caucasian population in the United States

The first signs of psoriatic arthritis usually occur between 40 and 50 years of age, but may strike at any age even children.

Males and females are affected equally. The skin disease psoriasis and the joint disease arthritis frequently appear separately, the skin disease precedes the arthritis in nearly 80% of patients. The arthritis, more rarely will precede the psoriasis in about 15% of patients, in some cases by over

20 years. Patients may have psoriasis for over 20 years before arthritis develops.

Psoriatic arthritis may more rarely become a systemic disease that can cause inflammation in body tissues other than the joints other and skin, including the eyes, heart, lungs, and kidneys and may be associated with Crohn's disease and ulcerative colitis. Inflammation in the spine is almost classical in psoriatic arthritis and frequently referred to as spondyloarthropathies.

The cause of psoriatic arthritis is currently unknown, but combinations of genetic and environmental factors are likely involved and changes in the immune system are important.

Symptoms of psoriatic arthritis

Psoriatic arthritis may affect just one or many joints. Signs and symptoms of psoriatic arthritis include pain in the affected joints, swelling in affected joints, heat, and redness that are warm to the toucan those joints. A pattern has been identified in which psoriatic arthritis typically occurs and most patients move from one pattern of psoriatic arthritis to another throughout the course of their disease.

This pattern is in five stages.

1. The mildest form of psoriatic arthritis is called asymmetric psoriatic arthritis and usually affects joints on only one side of the body or different joints on each side, which may include the hip, knee, ankle or wrist. When asymmetric arthritis occurs in the hands and feet, swelling and inflammation in the affected tendons may cause those fingers and toes to resemble small sausages called dactylitis.

2. Symmetric psoriatic arthritis, the second stage, usually affects four or more of the same joints but on both sides of the body. More women than men have symmetric psoriatic arthritis and the psoriasis associated with the condition tends to be more severe.

3. Distal interphalangeal joint predominant psoriatic arthritis is rare occurring mostly in men. This stage affects the small joints closest to the nails, the distal joints, in the fingers and toes.

4. This form of psoriatic arthritis, called spondylitis, causes inflammation in the spine as well as stiffness and inflammation in the neck, lower back or sacroiliac joints. Inflammation may occur where ligaments and tendons attach to the spine as well and over time tends to become increasingly painful and difficult.

5. A small percentage of people with psoriatic arthritis will develop arthritis mutilans, a severe, painful and disabling form of this disease. In time, arthritis mutilans gradually destroys the small bones in the hands, especially the fingers, leading to permanent deformity and disability.

Inflammation of the chest wall and of the cartilage that links the ribs to the breastbone may occur, causing severe chest pain, called costochondritis. Furthermore, psoriatic arthritis might cause inflammation in other organs, such as the eyes, lungs, and aorta. Inflammation in the colored portion of the eye, the iris, causes iritis, a painful condition aggravated by bright light as the iris opens and close. Inflammation in and around the lungs, pleuritis, causes chest pain, usually severe, especially with deep breathing;

this may result in shortness of breath. Inflammation of the aorta may cause leakage of the aortic valve, which may lead to heart failure. Also acne and nail changes are frequently seen with psoriatic arthritis and pitting and ridges are seen in finger and toe nails of up to 80% of patients.

Diagnosis of psoriatic arthritis

The diagnosis of psoriatic arthritis is made by assessment or the signs and symptoms and ruling out other causes of joint pain, such as osteoarthritis and rheumatoid arthritis. The tests that are used to help to distinguish psoriatic arthritis from other conditions include X-rays to help pinpoint changes in the joints occurring in psoriatic arthritis but not in other arthritic conditions, joint fluid tests for analysis in a laboratory, blood tests to checks your erythrocyte sedimentation rate which increases when inflammation is present and check for rheumatoid factor a protein made by the immune system that's often present in the blood of people with rheumatoid arthritis, but not in the blood of people with psoriatic arthritis. Nevertheless, most people are diagnosed with psoriasis before they begin experiencing the pain of psoriatic arthritis making the diagnosis easier

Treatments and drugs

No cure exists yet for psoriatic arthritis. Treatment is aimed to control inflammation in the affected joints in order to prevent joint pain and disability, usually accomplished with medications and, rarely, surgery.

Medications commonly used to treat psoriatic arthritis include the nonsteroidal anti-inflammatory drugs or NSAIDs such as aspirin and ibuprofen, which help control pain, swelling and morning stiffness. Corticosteroids might be recommended to control infrequent joint pain flares. Corticosteroids may be taken orally or they might be injected directly into painful joints providing almost immediate relief and improve range of motion and sometimes lasting for months.

Another class of drugs often used in treating psoriatic arthritis is disease-modifying anti-rheumatic drugs or DMARDs. Rather than just reducing pain and inflammation, these drugs help to limit the amount of joint damage that occurs in psoriatic arthritis. Examples of DMARDs include Sulfasalazine trade name Azulfidine, hydroxychloroquine and methotrexate.

Immunosuppressant medications act to suppress the immune system, which normally protects the body from harmful organisms, but in error attacks healthy tissue in people with psoriatic arthritis. Immunosuppressant drugs can have potentially dangerous side effects and usually are used for only the most severe cases of psoriatic arthritis. Because they suppress the immune system, these drugs can lead to anemia and an increased risk of serious infection and may cause liver and kidney problems.

Surgery is rarely performed for psoriatic arthritis but may be recommended in some form of joint operation when other treatments fail to relieve symptoms or maintain function. Replacement of hips or knee joints is rarely necessary. To maintain function and range of motion exercise programs can be done at home or with a physical therapist and are customized according to the disease and physical capabilities of each patient. These should include warm-up stretching, or other techniques, such as hot shower or heat applications helpful to relax muscles prior to exercise and ice application after the routine can help minimize post-exercise soreness and inflammation.

Exercises for arthritis are performed mainly for the purpose of strengthening and maintaining or improving joint range of motion.

CHAPTER 8

ANKYLOSING SPONDYLITIS

Ankylosing spondylitis is a form of chronic arthritic inflammation of the spine and the sacroiliac joints located in the low back where the sacrum or the bone directly above the tailbone meets the iliac bones at the back of the pelvis. The inflammation in these areas causes pain and stiffness in and around the spine from the neck to the tailbone. Over sufficient time, this chronic spinal inflammation, called spondylitis, can lead to a complete fusion of the vertebrae; this fusion is referred to as ankylosis and leads to loss of mobility of the spine.

Ankylosing spondylitis may also become a systemic rheumatic disease, in which case it can affect other tissues throughout the body. It can cause inflammation to other joints than the spine and other organs, such as the eyes, heart, lungs, and kidneys. several other arthritis conditions, such as psoriatic arthritis, reactive arthritis, and arthritis associated with Crohn's disease and ulcerative colitis share many features with ankylosing spondylitis They may also cause disease and inflammation in the spine, other joints, eyes, skin, mouth, and various organs. These symptom-related conditions are collectively referred to as spondyloarthropathies.

Ankylosing spondylitis affects all age groups, including young children. It appears two to three times more commonly in males than in females and in women; joints other than the spines are more frequently affected than in men.

The most common ages of onset of symptoms are in the second and third decades of life.

Ankylosing spondylitis is believed to be genetically inherited, and in nearly 90% of all patients with this disease are born with a common gene. However, this specific gene appears only to increase the tendency of developing Ankylosing spondylitis, so environmental factors are likely necessary for the disease to appear. In gene positive individuals having relatives with the disease, their risk of developing Ankylosing spondylitis rises to 12% or six times greater than for those without relatives having Ankylosing spondylitis.

Symptoms of Ankylosing spondylitis

The symptoms of ankylosing spondylitis reflect the inflammation of the spine, joints, and other organs involved in the patient. Fatigue becomes a common symptom associated to active inflammation. Inflammation of the spine causes pain and stiffness in the low back, upper buttock area, the remainder of the spine and neck. Onset of pain and stiffness is usually gradual and progressively worsens over several months. On rarer occasions, the onset may be rapid and quite intense. Pain and stiffness are often worse in the morning or after prolonged sedentary periods of inactivity. Activity usually eases the pain and stiffness, as will heat or a warm shower.

Some patients who have chronic and severe inflammation of the spine can develop a complete bony fusion of the spine called ankylosis; once fused, the pain in the spine disappears however; the patient has a complete loss of spine mobility. These completely fused spines are fragile, brittle and vulnerable to fracture. The lower neck or cervical spine is the most common area for such fractures.

Chronic ankylosing spondylitis may cause forward curvature of the thoracic spine, severely limiting breathing motion and can also affect the areas where ribs attach to the upper spine, further limiting lung capacity. To further reduce breathing and lung function ankylosing spondylitis can cause inflammation and scarring of the lungs, causing severe coughing and shortness of breath, especially during exercise or infections. In some cases, the small joints of the toes can become inflamed and sausage shaped. Inflammation may occur in the cartilage around the breastbone causing costochondritis as well as in the tendons attaching the muscles to the bone causing tendonitis

Diagnosis

The diagnosis of ankylosing spondylitis is made by evaluating the patient's symptom history, a physical examination, x-ray findings, and blood tests. The examination should show signs of inflammation and decreased range of motion in the affected joints, particularly in the spine where flexibility of the low back and/or neck may be decreased. There might be pain and tenderness of the sacroiliac joints and the expansion of the chest with full breathing may be limited by rigidity of the chest wall.

X-ray and laboratory findings provide clues to nail down the diagnosis. Abnormalities will show in x-rays of the spine. The presence of the blood test will show the genetic marker, HLA-B27 gene in a high percentage of cases. Other blood tests may provide evidence of inflammation via the sedimentation rate indicator for inflammation throughout the body. Urinalysis should be done to look for accompanying abnormalities of the kidney and to exclude kidney conditions that could mimics ankylosing spondylitis. Patients should also evaluated for symptoms and signs of other related spondyloarthropathies, such as psoriasis, venereal disease, Reiter's disease, and inflammatory bowel disease such as ulcerative colitis or Crohn's disease.

Treatment

The treatments for ankylosing spondylitis involve the use of medications to reduce inflammation and to suppress immunity. Physical therapy and exercise are used to increase and restore function and help improve posture, spine mobility, and lung capacity. Aspirin and other NSAIDs are commonly used to decrease pain and stiffness of the affected joints. These NSAIDs include indomethacin, tolmetin, sulindac, naproxen and diclofenac. The additions of medications that suppress the body's immune system are considered in more severe cases. These medications may bring about long-term reduction of inflammation. Oral or injectable corticosteroids are potent anti-inflammatory agents and can effectively control spondylitis and other inflammations in the body; however, corticosteroids can have serious side effects when used on a long-term basis. These side effects may include cataracts, thinning of the skin and bones, severe bruising, infections, diabetes, and destruction of large joints, such as the hips and knees.

Physical therapy for ankylosing spondylitis includes exercises to maintain proper posture, preserve, and increase function such as deep breathing for lung expansion and stretching exercises to improve spine and joint mobility. Exercise programs should be customized for the individual patient. Swimming is ideal, as it avoids jarring impact on the spine. Aerobic exercise is usually encouraged to promote full expansion of breathing muscles and joints.

Inflammation and diseases in other organs are treated as indicated for those specific problems. This may require consultation and treatment of various other specialties such as ophthalmology, cardiology, gastroenterology or others.

Cigarette smoking is especially and strongly discouraged in patients with ankylosing spondylitis because it accelerates lung scarring and breathing difficulties.

Occasionally, patients with ankylosing spondylitis may require oxygen supplementation and medications to improve breathing. Smoking cessation in this disease is so important that we have included the **Quit Smoking Now™** program free in the appendix of this book.

In long standing and sever disease where the hip, knee joints and spine are severely damaged orthopedic surgery may be required.

CHAPTER 9

REITER'S SYNDROME OR REACTIVE ARTHRITIS

Reactive arthritis is a chronic and features three conditions, which are inflamed joints, inflammation of the eyes or conjunctivitis and inflammation of the genital, urinary, or gastrointestinal systems. This arthritic disease is called reactive arthritis because it is thought to involve an immune system reacting to the presence of bacterial infections in the genital, urinary, or gastrointestinal systems, the immune system then attacking the joints. It appears that in these cases the immune systems genetically react aberrantly when these areas are exposed to certain bacteria. This aberrant reaction of the immune system leads may lead to confusion in diagnosis as presentation of the arthritis or eye inflammation may occur long after the initial infection. Reactive arthritis has been referred to as Reiter syndrome named after Dr. Hans Reiter who first described it. Reactive arthritis most frequently first occurs in patients during their 30s or 40s, however it may occur at any age.

Reactive arthritis is a systemic rheumatic disease meaning it can affect other organs than just the joints, causing inflammation in organ systems such as the eyes, mouth, skin, kidneys, heart, and lungs. Reactive arthritis that occurs after genital infection, often venereal occurs more frequently in males while that which develops after a bowel infection occurs in equal frequency in males and females. Reactive arthritis shares numerous features with other arthritic conditions including psoriatic arthritis, ankylosing spondylitis, and arthritis associated with Crohn's disease and ulcerative colitis. Since each of these arthritic conditions may cause similar disease and inflammation in the spine and other joints, eyes, skin, mouth, and various organs they are collectively referred to as spondyloarthropathies.

Reactive arthritis is felt at least in part to be genetic and there are certain genetic markers that are more frequently found in patients with reactive arthritis than in the general population; however even in these patients who have the genetic markers that predisposes them to the development of reactive arthritis, exposure to certain infections seem required to trigger the onset of this disease. Usually the arthritis and conjunctivitis develops one to three weeks after the onset of the bacterial infection.

Symptoms of reactive arthritis

A common pneumonic used by medical students to remember reactive arthritis is, "Can't see, can't pee, can't bend the knee!"

Classically the joints that usually become inflamed in reactive arthritis are the knees, ankles, feet, and wrists. Joints involvement is usually asymmetric, meaning one side of the body or the other is affected, rather than both sides simultaneously. This inflammation leads to stiffness, severe pain, swelling, warmth, and redness of the joints involved. Often patients will develop inflammation of fingers or toes, which may give the appearance of a sausage like digit. As mentioned above, reactive arthritis can be associated with inflammation of the spine, leading to stiffness and pain in the back or neck as is characteristic of all the spondyloarthropathies.

Cartilages may become inflamed, especially around the sternum or breastbone where the ribs bones meet at the front of the chest, a condition called costochondritis, which can cause difficulties with respiration. In reactive arthritis, the tendon insertion points where muscles attach to the bones can become inflamed causing tendonitis and painful movement of the affected joint. .

When organ systems become inflamed, they cause symptoms of pain and irritation in the eyes, genitals, urinary tract including the urethra, bladder and prostate gland. In addition, the skin, mouth lining, large bowel, and the aorta may become involved along with the gastrointestinal system. Inflammation of the white portion of the eye or conjunctivitis and the iris of the eye or iritis is frequently seen early in reactive arthritis. Iritis can be very painful especially when looking toward bright lights while conjunctivitis may be relatively painless. Urinary tract inflammation may be associated with burning on urination and pus drainage from the penis. The skin of the penis may become inflamed and sometimes peel. The bladder and prostate gland may become inflamed, leading to an urgency to urinate and cause a transient incontinence.

When the gastrointestinal system is involved, the mouth may show ulcerations in the mucous membrane and on the tongue. These lesions are often painless and may go unnoticed by the patient. Inflammation of the large bowel or colitis will usually cause severe diarrhea with pus or blood in the stool.

Inflammation of the aorta is seen in a small percentage of patients who have reactive arthritis and may lead to failure of the aortic valve of the heart, which may cause heart failure. If the electrical conducting pathways of the heart become scarred in reactive arthritis, it can lead to serious irregular heartbeats or arrhythmias often requiring a pacemaker to regulate the heartbeat.

Often the skin on the palms of the hands and the soles of the feet develop tiny blisters and the affected skin may peel to mimic psoriasis. These are referred to as keratoderma blennorrhagica.

Diagnosis of reactive arthritis

The diagnosis of reactive arthritis is often missed early on because of the lag time between the various symptoms and organ system involvements. Furthermore, there is no single lab test able to diagnose reactive arthritis. Instead, reactive arthritis is usually diagnosed by recognition of the combination of arthritis with inflammation of the eyes, and the genital, urinary, or gastrointestinal systems. A thorough medical history noting the time course of infection in the eyes, genital or urinary tracts, or bowel in relation to recent arthritis symptoms give the first and best clues to diagnosis. Stiffness and pain in joints should be monitored. Blood tests such as a sedimentation rate may be obtained to document the presence of inflammation in the body but are not at all specific for reactive arthritis. To help differentiate reactive arthritis the rheumatoid factor, which is typically present in rheumatoid arthritis, is usually negative in reactive arthritis. The HLA-B27 gene marker blood test may be somewhat helpful. Stool cultures should be obtained in cases involving the gastrointestinal tract to detect the presence of infections in the bowel. Similarly, urinalysis and culture of the urine should be examined to detect bacterial infection in the urinary tract. The prostate gland, which can also be inflamed in a patient with reactive arthritis, should be examined for tenderness.

X-rays of the spine and other joints might reveal typical changes of inflammation in affected areas but usually not until later in the disease and these changes are not specific to reactive arthritis.

Treatment

Treatment of reactive arthritis varies with systems of the body that are involved. The joint pains and inflammation are usually treated initially with nonsteroidal anti-inflammatory drugs or the NSAIDs, including aspirin, indomethacin, tolmetin, sulindac, piroxicam and others. Corticosteroids, such as prednisone, may be used to reduce inflammation in the short-term treatment of inflammation in reactive arthritis. These may be given by mouth or by local injection into the affected joints.

For the more aggressive joint inflammation, medications that suppress the immune system are used. Sulfasalazine, trade name Azulfadine, has been shown to be effective in some patients with persistent reactive arthritis. When bacteria are discovered in the bowel or urine, treatment with antibiotics specific for those bacterial infections are given.

Eye inflammation is usually alleviated with anti-inflammatory eye drops, but patients with severe iritis require local injections of cortisone into the eye to prevent damaging inflammation, which can lead to blindness.

CHAPTER 10

ADULT STILL'S DISEASE

Adult Still's disease or ASD is an inflammatory condition in which the patient may experience daily spiking fevers, with achy or swollen joints and develops a salmon-pink rash on the body. The disorder is rare. Though not common, ASD needs to be taken seriously as a potentially debilitating disease that may cause serious damage and problems to the joints, heart, lungs, liver and spleen. While a mild form of the disease responds quite well to NSAID drugs, a severe, chronic form that is more difficult to treat can cause long term pain and disability or even death.

Adult Still's Disease gets its name from Dr. George Still, a British pediatrician, who first identified the childhood form of the disease.

Though rare, it predominantly affects young adults between 16 and 35. As it progresses, Adult Still's disease may lead to chronic arthritis and other complications.

Symptoms
Patients with Adult Still's disease experience a

combination of signs and symptoms, which may include a daily fever of at least 102 F for up to a week or longer usually peaking in the late afternoon or early evening. Between peaks, the temperature will tend to return to normal. A salmon-pink either bumpy or flat rash may come and go with the fever. The rash usually appears on the trunk of the body and arms or legs. Achy and swollen joints appear especially those of the knees, wrists, ankles and elbows. They become stiff, painful and inflamed. Usually, the joint discomfort lasts two or more weeks. Muscular pain usually ebbs and flows with the fever and may be severe enough to disrupt your daily activities. Other signs and symptoms may include sore throat, swollen lymph nodes in your neck and an enlarged liver or spleen.

Causes

Although it is not certain what causes Adult Still's disease, it appears to be triggered by a viral or bacterial infection. The rubella or German Measles virus has been detected in many people with ASD cases and researchers have also found some association between mumps, parainfluenza, and other viruses. A genetic immune disorder and hormonal factors may also be influential. It appears that pregnant women are slightly more likely to come down with ASD. This disease seems to affect both sexes equally. Age seems to be the main risk factor for Adult Still's disease, with the incidence in adults peaking once from 15 to 25 years of age and again from 36 to 46 years

Tests and diagnosis

At present there's no single test used to diagnose Adult Still's disease. Because the signs and symptoms of Adult

Still's disease may mimic those of several other conditions, like mononucleosis, lymphoma or other rheumatic diseases diagnosis may be based on a number of factors.

Signs and symptoms.

A thorough history and physical exam may lead to the suspicion of Adult Still's disease if they reveal a high fever, swollen joints and a salmon-pink rash. Swollen lymph nodes and a sore throat may also be an added clue.

Imaging tests

Inflammation of the lining of the heart or lungs may be detected by an echocardiogram and X-rays of your joints may show changes in your wrists, spine, foot or finger joints, while a computerized tomography or CT scan or ultrasound may indicate that your liver or spleen is enlarged.

Blood tests

Blood tests may give an indication that you have Adult Still's disease. Typically, the number of white blood cells and platelets are high, while the red blood cell count is often low revealing anemia. The erythrocyte sedimentation rate can reveal inflammation in the body. In addition, liver function tests should be run to determine how well your liver is performing. In cases of Adult Still's disease, levels of certain liver enzymes may be elevated.

Complications

Complications from adult Still's disease may arise from chronic inflammation of your body organs and joints. These can be seriously debilitating and in rare cases fatal.

Joint destruction

Chronic and long-term inflammation can permanently damage joints; most commonly involved joints are wrists, neck, feet, fingers, hips and knee joints. In severe cases, joint replacement surgery may be necessary in hips or knee joints.

Inflammation of the heart

Adult Still's disease may lead to inflammation of the covering of your heart known as pericarditis, or of the muscular portion of your heart called myocarditis.

Excess fluid around the lungs

Inflammation around and in the lungs may cause an excess of fluid to build up in the space that surrounds your lungs.

Treatment

The most widely used treatment for ASD and its symptoms is non-steroidal anti-inflammatory drugs, the NSAIDs. Statistically, 20-25% of ASD sufferers improve by treatment with NSAIDs. NSAIDs are may be taken for 1 to 3 months after the symptoms are gone. In severe cases, doctors may also prescribe corticosteroids to address heart, blood, and other life-threatening problems that ASD may cause. Anti-TNF therapy, aimed at a component of the immune system, may be an additional therapy.

Some ASD sufferers do not respond well to NSAIDs and go on to develop the chronic form of the disease. Because corticosteroids have serious side effects, they should not be used to treat ASD over a period of years. Instead, doctors may prescribe drugs such as methotrexate,

IM gold, D-penicillamine, hydroxychloroquine and azathioprine. Cyclophosphamide is reserved only for the most difficult cases.

In addition to medications, there are a few ways to help you make the most of your health if you have Adult Still's disease. The course of this disease can be improved by complying with your physician's order by taking medications as recommends, regularly and for as long as prescribed, to control inflammation, which helps reduce the risk of complications and permanent joint and organ damage.

Exercise is extremely important to maintain joint and muscle function. Keep moving even if you don't feel up to a workout when your joints ache; exercising can maintain your range of motion and relieve pain and stiffness.

CHAPTER 11

VIRAL ARTHRITIS

The number of patients diagnosed with acute viral arthritis is low because of its late presentation following its triggering infection. Viruses cause infection and are in rare instances triggering factors in the development of rheumatic arthritic diseases. Viral infections are dependent on host factors, which include age, sex, genetic background, infection history, and the body's immune response. In some rare cases, a viral infection may cause an autoimmune response leading to joint involvement known as viral arthritis. In the great majority of such cases the disease is short lived and transient. Viral arthritis occurs worldwide, but precise incidence rates of viral arthritis are unknown. The major morbidity of viral arthritis is dysfunctional joints. The mortality rate depends on the type of virus and duration of infection. Though the incidence is greater in Africa and Asia, there appears to be no racial or ethnic predilection recognized. This disease may affect children as well as adults.

In the United States, patients with the most common viral arthritis generally present with a rash and symmetrical small joint involvement, although different patterns of joint and soft tissue involvement present with different types of viral infections. Typically, the viral arthritis occurs during the viral prodromes when the characteristic rash arises. In some instances, there may be a low-grade fever but usually the viral symptoms occur after the arthritis. In virtually all instances, the arthritis associated with viral infections is nondestructive and does not lead to any known form of chronic disease.

The viral symptoms vary with the type of viral infection involved. For example, parvovirus B19 is a small virus, which may be responsible for causing approximately 12% of the cases of sudden-onset polyarticular arthritis, particularly in adults with frequent exposures to children, like schoolteachers and pediatric nurses. Outbreaks commonly occur in late winter and spring, but the condition can be observed during summer and fall, sporadic cases occurring throughout the year.

In children, the clinical features include flu-like symptoms of fever, headache, sore throat, cough, anorexia, vomiting, diarrhea and arthralgia. A bright red rash is typically noted, especially on the face giving a characterized "slapped cheeks" appearance. In children, joint symptoms are rare appearing in 5 to 10% of cases.

The clinical features in adults differ in that joint symptoms occur in up to 60% of cases. This is more often an arthralgia rather than frank arthritis. This arthralgia is usually self-limited; symmetrical; and in the peripheral small joints of the hands, wrists, knees, and ankle joints, with morning stiffness and swelling. However, in adults, rash is rare

Hepatitis A virus accounts infection for 10% to14% of cases of viral arthritis. Arthralgia and skin rash occur during the acute phase. Transmission is via the fecal-oral route. The hepatitis B virus or HBV infection accounts for 20% to 25% of cases of viral arthritis. Transmission of HBV can be parenteral or sexual. The hepatitis C virus or HCV infection occurs worldwide. It is a rapidly progressive with acute arthralgia but rarely causing true arthritis. Its distribution usually affects the hands, wrists, shoulders, knees, and hips. Myalgia is very common. Several recent reports have described a possible association between fibromyalgia and HCV infection. Transmission of HVC can be parenteral or, uncommonly sexual.

There are literally dozens of viruses that may be responsible for triggering viral arthritis and fortunately, it is rare for this disease to cause any permanent damage to joints. Probably in most cases, it is shrugged of as, "You've got the flu bug, take aspirin and go to bed…"

Treatment

In general, the great majority of cases of viral arthritis are mild and patients require only symptomatic treatment with analgesics or nonsteroidal anti-inflammatory drugs the NSAIDs. Occasionally, a brief course of low-dose prednisone may be required.

For parvovirus B19, the treatment is symptomatic with analgesics and NSAIDs. In very rare severe cases, aspiration of fluid from the affected joint may relieve pain.

Hepatitis A virus: Treatment is also usually only symptomatic with analgesics and NSAIDs. Most important in this disease is prophylaxis for contacts with other people and family members.

Hepatitis B virus patients with acute icteric HBV infection recover without residual injury or chronic hepatitis. Focus management of acute HBV infection on avoidance of further hepatic injury and prophylaxis of contacts.

Hepatitis C virus patients may require administration of interferon alfa-2b and combination therapy with ribavirin is recommended and has been shown to yield better response rates. Corticosteroids and cyclophosphamide may be required initially for patients with more active, severe vasculitic complications.

It is very rare for viral arthritis infections to cause any permanent damage to the joints.

Chapter 12

Gonococcal Arthritis

Gonococcal arthritis sometimes called disseminated gonococcal infection or simply DGI, is basically inflammation of a joint and usually just one joint, secondary to a gonorrhea infection. Gonorrhea is certainly not the only bacteria to cause an infected joint and arthritis, but it is by far the most common.

Gonococcal arthritis is a bacterial infection of a joint that occurs in people who have gonorrhea and it affects women four times more often than men and is most commonly found among sexually active adolescent girls.

There are two forms of gonococcal arthritis; one involves skin rashes and multiple joints, usually the large joints such as the knees, wrists and ankles, while the second and less common form involves disseminated gonococcemia, which leads to infection of a single joint.

Symptoms

The symptoms of gonococcal arthritis include fever, lower abdominal pain, migrating joint pain lasting from one to four days, pain in the hands or wrists due to tendonitis, pain and burning on urination often with discharge, single joint pain and a skin rash that is flat, pink to red, or may appear purple and may contain puss.

Diagnosis

The diagnosis of Gonococcal arthritis is easily made with a series of laboratory exams. Blood cultures should be taken and evaluated in all cases of suspected Gonococcal arthritis. Further tests should be done to check for a gonorrhea infection; this involves the taking samples of tissue, stool, joint fluids, or other body material and sending them to a lab for examination under a microscope and cultures. Such tests include cervical swab gram stains, culture of joint fluid aspirate, joint fluid gram stain, and a throat culture

Treatment

All gonorrhea infections must be treated. There are two aspects to treating any sexually transmitted disease; the first is to cure the infection and the second is to seek out, test, and treat all sexual contacts of the infected person to prevent further spread of the STD or sexually transmitted disease. The recommended treatment is with the drugs Ceftriaxone or Cefixime and in addition treatment for Chlamydia if it can't be ruled out. A follow-up exam is advised at seven days after treatment to recheck blood tests and confirm the cure of infection. With proper treatment symptoms usually improve within one to two days and a full recovery can be expected; however untreated, this condition may lead to persistent joint pain and damage.

Septic arthritis, Blastomycosis and fungal infectious arthritis

There are many bacterial, fungal and microscopic organisms that may on rarer occasions cause a septic arthritis other than Gonococcal arthritis. There are various routs by which these organisms may enter a joint or joints to infect them. Most are usually monoarthritic and treatment of each is dependent on their individual drug sensitivity. If left untreated they may lead to sever damage to the affected joints.

CHAPTER 13

FIBROMYALGIA

Fibromyalgia is a chronic arthritic condition characterized by widespread aching and pain in the muscles, ligaments and tendons and multiple joints and accompanied by debilitating fatigue and multiple tender points on the body where even the slightest pressure may causes pain. Fibromyalgia is more common in women than in men.

The intensity of symptoms may vary from time to time, but they will probably never disappear completely. Fibromyalgia is not progressive or life threatening.

Symptoms

Signs and symptoms of fibromyalgia vary considerably from patient to patient depending on the triggering causes, which can include, stress, physical activity or even the time of day. The common signs and symptoms include widespread pain, fatigue and sleep disturbances, irritable bowel syndrome, headache and facial pain and heightened sensory sensitivity. Fibromyalgia patients suffer pain in specific areas of the body when pressure is applied, in the back of your head, upper back and neck, upper chest, elbows, hips and knees. The pain often persists for months at a time and is usually accompanied by stiffness.

Patients with fibromyalgia may wake up tired and un-refreshed even though they seem to get sufficient of sleep. People with fibromyalgia appear to miss the deep restorative stage of sleep. Nighttime muscle spasms in their legs and restless legs syndrome also seem to be associated with fibromyalgia.

The constipation, diarrhea, abdominal pain and bloating associated with irritable bowel syndrome are commonly present in people suffering fibromyalgia. Patients who have fibromyalgia also frequently suffer headaches and facial pain that may be accompanied tenderness or stiffness in their neck and shoulders. Temporomandibular joint or TMJ dysfunction, which affects the jaw joints and surrounding muscles with severe pain, may also appear in people with fibromyalgia. Furthermore, patients with fibromyalgia may be hypersensitive to odors, noises, bright lights and touch.

Other common signs and symptoms include depression, numbness or tingling sensations in the hands and feet or paresthesias, difficulty concentrating and focusing, mood swings, chest pain, dry eyes, skin and mouth, painful menstrual periods, vertigo and anxiety

Causes of Fibromyalgia

Doctors and researchers do not know what causes fibromyalgia, but the current thinking centers on a "central sensitization" theory. This theory considers that people with fibromyalgia have a lower threshold for pain because of the increased sensitivity in the brain to pain signals.

Researchers believe repeated nerve stimulation and impulses actually cause the brains of fibromyalgia patients to change. This change may be due to an abnormal increase in levels of certain chemicals, the neurotransmitters, in the brain that signal pain excessive pain. In addition, the brain's pain receptors seem overreact to pain signals. What actually initiates this process of central nervous system hyper-sensitization is not known or understood.

It is quite likely that a number of factors contribute to the development of fibromyalgia. These causes of fibromyalgia might be related to sleep disturbances, injury, infection, abnormalities of the autonomic or sympathetic nervous system and changes in muscle metabolism. Psychological stress and hormonal changes may also be possible causes or triggers of fibromyalgia.

Risk factors

Fibromyalgia occurs more often in women than in men and tends to develop during early and middle adulthood, but it has on rare occasion occurred in children as well as in older adults.

It is unclear whether sleeping difficulties are a cause or the result of fibromyalgia, but it appears that people with sleep disorders, like nighttime muscle spasms in their legs, restless legs syndrome or sleep apnea, may also develop fibromyalgia. You may be more likely to develop fibromyalgia if a relative also has the condition pointing to a possible genetic predisposition. Having a rheumatic disease, such as rheumatoid arthritis, lupus or ankylosing spondylitis, may cause a person to be more likely to have fibromyalgia.

Diagnosis

Fibromyalgia is a difficult diagnosis to make because there isn't a specific diagnostic laboratory test. The fact is that it is most often a diagnosis by process of elimination. Before making a diagnosis of fibromyalgia doctors usually, go through numerous medical tests, including blood tests and X-rays, only to have the results come back normal. These tests usually help to rule out other conditions, such as rheumatoid arthritis, lupus and multiple sclerosis, but they cannot confirm fibromyalgia.

Finally, the American College of Rheumatology has established general guidelines for fibromyalgia study and diagnosis. Following these guidelines, to be diagnosed with fibromyalgia the patient must have experienced widespread aching and pain for at minimum three months and have at least eleven locations on the body that are abnormally tender under relatively mild, firm pressure. Of particular interest are specific points of tenderness on the patient's head, upper body. However not all doctors agree with these guidelines feeling that these criteria are far too rigid.

Treatments

The main emphasis in treating fibromyalgia is toward minimizing symptoms and improving general health and function. This care generally includes medication and self-care.

Medications

Medications utilized most often are chosen to reduce the pain of fibromyalgia and improve, function, sleep and psychological well-being.

Analgesics used for pain relief include acetaminophen or Tylenol, ibuprofen, aspirin, indomethacin and others NSAIDs. These it is hoped may ease the pain and stiffness caused by fibromyalgia. However, its effectiveness varies. However, NSAIDs have not proved to be effective in managing the pain in fibromyalgia when taken by themselves. Antidepressants are frequently prescribed such promote sleep and help if the patient is also experiencing depression. A newer class of antidepressants known as serotonin and nor-epinephrine reuptake inhibitors, which regulate two brain chemicals involved in the transition pain signals show some promise.

Taking muscle relaxants at bedtime may help treat muscle pain and spasms. Pregabalin, a seizure medication that seems to reduce pain and improve function in people with fibromyalgia and is the first medication the Federal Drug Administration has approved to treat fibromyalgia. The side effects of pregabalin include vertigo, insomnia, difficulty focusing and concentrating, blurred vision, weight gain, dry mouth, and swelling of the hands and feet. Prescription sleeping pills, such as Ambien may provide benefits but many doctors advise against long-term use of these drugs. Frequently, using sleeping pills tends to create even more sleeping problems for some people.

Doctors rarely recommend narcotics for treating fibromyalgia because of the potential for dependence and addiction. The corticosteroids have not been shown to be effective in treating fibromyalgia.

Cognitive behavior therapy may be utilized to restore and strengthen confidence in a patient's abilities and for dealing with stressful situations.

Treatment programs usually combine a number of modalities to improve symptoms, pain relief and restoration of function. Programs may combine relaxation techniques, biofeedback and pain clinic consultation.

Other critical aspects in the management of fibromyalgia include reduction of stress and the avoidance of overexertion. Patients must get sufficient sleep because fatigue is one of the main characteristics of fibromyalgia. Exercising regularly and often on a regular schedule generally decreases symptoms. The best exercises include walking, swimming, biking and water aerobics. Eat a healthy diet that limits caffeine intake and offers good nutrition.

Many fibromyalgia patients have turned to alternative medication as a complementary and treatment for pain and stress management, such as meditation, yoga, acupuncture and chiropractic. Their use has become popular, especially with people who have chronic illnesses, such as fibromyalgia. These treatments appear to safely relieve stress and reduce pain, and are gaining acceptance in mainstream medicine.

CHAPTER 14

TERTIARY LYME DISEASE

Lime disease was not note until recent years. It is still relatively rare and is its chronic form is known by several names including Tertiary Lyme disease, Stage 3 Lyme disease and late persistent Lyme disease. It is a late and chronic stage of an inflammatory disease caused by Borrelia burgdorferi bacteria. Lyme disease is transmitted by the bite of a deer tick, but Tertiary Lyme disease occurs months to years after the initial infection with Lyme disease. Lyme disease is not contagious from person to person.

Symptoms

Chronic persistent Lyme disease may affect the skin, brain and nervous system, as well as muscles, bones, cartilage and joints. Its symptoms include: chronic arthritis, joint inflammation in the knees and other large joints, memory loss, mood swings and changes, sleep disorders, abnormal sensitivity to light or photophobia, confusion and disorientation and numbness and tingling

Diagnosis

Fortunately there is and ELISA for Lyme disease test making the diagnosis simpler. It is a blood test to check for antibodies to the bacteria that cause Lyme disease. Another test, the Western blot test is done to confirm ELISA results. A spinal tap will also be abnormal if the patient has central nervous system symptoms related to Lyme disease.

Treatment
Antibiotics are given to fight the infection and NSAIDs can be used to relieve the arthritic symptoms. The arthritis symptoms may not get better with treatment but the other symptoms should improve with treatment. A person may rarely continue to have symptoms that will continue to interfere with daily life or activities. This is often labelled post-Lyme disease syndrome and unfortunately, there is no effective treatment for these persistent symptoms. Arthritis symptoms may become chronic.

Prevention

Prevention methods are the best course in Lyme disease. When hiking in wooded or grassy areas spray all exposed skin and clothing with insect repellent.

Wear light-colored clothing making it easier to spot ticks. Wear long-sleeved shirts and long pants with the cuffs tucked into shoes or socks and wear high, preferably rubber boots. Most importantly, check yourself, your fellow hikers and your pets frequently during and after your hike. The ticks that carry Lyme disease are extremely small and hard to see. After returning home, remove your clothes and thoroughly inspect all skin surface areas, including your scalp. Early diagnosis and appropriate antibiotic treatment for essential for Lyme disease and is the most effective way to prevent tertiary Lyme disease. Carefully examine children.

Chapter 15

Tuberculosis Arthritis

Tuberculosis arthritis is infection of one or more joints by the Mycobacterium tuberculosis that leads to a bacterial aseptic arthritis. It is usually a monoarthritis of a hip or knee and, less commonly an ankle, elbow, wrist or shoulder. Tuberculosis infections may spread to bone in childhood when the long bones are growing and remain latent at these sites to re-activate years later, particularly in the elderly and in immuno-suppressed patients.

Diagnosis
The most common symptoms of tuberculosis arthritis are pain and stiffness which may in a few cases lead to paralysis of the lower limbs. Tubercular arthritis is usually a monoarthritis affecting primarily the hip or knee and less commonly the ankle, elbow, wrist and shoulder. **The systemic signs and symptoms of TB may also be present. Synovial fluid and synovial biopsies can be taken through arthroscopy to be studied microscopically. Culture of the biopsy material may be positive for the acid-fast TB bacilli even when synovial fluid is negative. Tuberculin skin tests may**

also be positive. Radiographs can show joint space narrowing, bony erosion and bony fragmentation.

Treatment

Treatment of Tuberculosis arthritis is by drainage of abscesses and immobilisation of the affected joints. The normal treatment also includes a six-month course of anti-Tuberculosis drugs. All treatments should be supervised by a physician with special and full training in the management of TB and with direct access to a TB nurse or health visitor. The type of isolation that will be required should be made by a TB specialist in consultation with an Infection Control Doctor to determine the infectiousness of the patient.

Treatment will also depend on whether the infection is active or latent, if. HIV is present, how much close contacts might be with patients with active infection and other high-risk groups such as IV drug users

CHAPTER 16

EXERCISES

This chapter is adapted from the book. "The Second Half Begins at Fifty... your longevity handbook" by Othniel Seiden, MD & Jane L. Bilett, PhD, see: www.BoomerBookSeries.com

Walking is the best aerobic exercise in which you can participate. You might at this point ask, "What is an *aerobic* exercise?" *Aerobic* means "with air" and refers to an activity that can be sustained without getting breathless ... as opposed to *anaerobic*, which creates an oxygen debt and its resulting breathlessness. Aerobic exercise, as opposed to anaerobic exercise, utilizes maximum oxygen. It works the heart and lungs for longer periods at a time than anaerobic. Anaerobic tend to work muscles against resistance for short spurts of time and uses minimum amounts of oxygen.

For arthritis patients an ideal program will utilize both aerobic and anaerobic exercises. The main goals an arthritis exercise program is to maintain mobility and function, maintain, and build strength in affected

joints.

Decide with your physician what your beginning level of exercise should be. If in doubt, start out with a minimal walk. Do what you know you can do even if it is only a few steps. If you do it with more ease than you expected, then add a few more steps with each walk you take. Even if you are just getting out of a sick bed and your walks are only a few feet, do them as often in the day as you can. Your walking program will progress at a much faster pace than you can imagine. Until you can walk for twenty minutes without a stop, do not feel you have to push yourself too far beyond comfort. The important thing is to make each walk a little further and/or a little faster than the last. In addition, walk every day. Make it part of your daily routine, preferably at the same time each day. It has to be scheduled to give it its proper priority among all the other things you do each day. In fact, it has to be at the very top of your priorities. Realize, *any day you do not find time to exercise walk you're saying everything you do that day is more important than your health!* Your health is your most important asset.

1. You will feel better all over with fewer aches and pains. When something does bother you, you'll bounce back quicker. You will probably have fewer "down days."
2. You will look far better, having more muscle tone throughout your entire body. You may not lose much weight, but you will have less fat and look trimmer.
3. You will be happier, more confident, have more energy and interests. Your friends and family will notice.

4. You will sleep better, deeper, more soundly.
5. You will find your joints are more supple, limber, and less subject to pain, injury and stiffness. Movement will be more fluid and easier.
6. You will think better, clearer and more creatively because of the improved circulation to your brain. This will influence the efficiency with which you do your job.
7. You will want to get out and do things you thought you'd never be interested in again. You will want to get out and do things.
8. You will enjoy friends and relatives a lot more and they will enjoy you. All your relationships should improve.
9. You will stop feeling sorry for yourself and may well want to help others achieve your state of health and happiness for themselves.
10. You will start looking for and setting new goals for yourself.
11. You will start thinking of your bright future instead of living in the past ... realizing that your life is still very much in front of you.

So get up right now and take your first steps toward that new life in front of you!

A lot has been written about stretching and warming up before you exercise. I feel the best warm up for walking is walking. Spend the first four or five minutes of your walk gradually working up to your best exercise pace. Start out at a comfortable walk, gradually increase your stride, and speed until you fall into a brisk rhythm that is adequate to give you a good cardiovascular workout.

More important than the warm up to your walk is an

adequate cool down period at the end of your walk. *Never, never* just stop after you've been walking at your ideal exercise pulse rate or faster without cooling down with a slower walk. Reduce you speed and continue to walk until your pulse is slowed to under your minimal exercise rate or less than 100, whichever is lower.

Then if you want to do some stretching exercises, do them after your workout. It is amazing how often people injure themselves by overstretching while their muscles are cold and tight before their workout. If you start your walk slow and easy and build up your pace, the muscles will warm up and limber safely. Then do your stretching after the vigorous workout. You will get all the benefits of stretching without the danger of injury. Furthermore, the post exercise stretching will keep you from getting stiff and painful muscles and joints after too vigorous a workout.

What about other sports … and what if you can't walk?

As for those few of you who can't walk due to a real physical handicap, the same principles apply. You must find an activity that will keep your joints mobile, functional and strong. Consider swimming, rowing or bicycling on a stationary rowing machine or bike or other water exercises such as pool aerobics, or just walk back and forth in a pool, trying to increase your speed and distance. You may find that these exercises will improve your condition to where you will be able to work into a walking program after all.

For those of you confined to a wheel chair, 45 minutes to an hour of wheeling yourself around a park is an ideal workout. Begin the same as recommended for the walking program, an easy spin at first, gradually adding to your time and distance and then adding to your speed until your working at your ideal exercise pulse rate for 45 minutes to an hour.

If you are bedridden or otherwise confined by your physical health, ask your physician about a physical therapy consultation to determine your true potential and how to reach it. There are very few who can do no exercise, but for those few, you can still maximize your fitness and life span by following the other lifestyle changes recommended in this book.

As for other exercises and sports activities, they are great if you enjoy them, but they do not replace your joint program. You should participate in as many exercise or athletic activities as you enjoy, over and above your joint improvement program. It is a good idea to have some other exercises available to you for those days when you can't walk because of inclement weather or some other preventing problem. Swimming, stationary biking or rowing are all ideal. All are good aerobic, low impact activities.

Such activities as tennis, racquet ball, baseball, weight lifting and training or body building, are anaerobic and wonderful activities, if you enjoy them, but remember they do not take the place of your joint improvement program and must be done in addition to your joint program.

Golf and bowling are great social and stress reducing activities and help keep your joints limber. Again, if you enjoy them, participate in them in addition to your joint program.

A special note about weight lifting and bodybuilding; both of these activities put special stresses on the heart and vascular system, which may have a detrimental effect on some cardiovascular conditions. Be sure to get a clearance and limitation of these activities from your cardiologist or cardiovascular surgeon!

In addition, do not forget that daily chores are also excellent joint improvers and Caloric burners. Don't farm them out to others to benefit from the activities. Do your own gardening, yard work, minor repairing whenever possible. Below is a list of Calorie expenditures for various activities. Just sitting on the couch burns few Calories.

Exercise Calorie Burners by Various Activities

This table will give you a rough idea of how many calories you may be burning at various activities when performed for 30 minutes. The Caloric expenditure listed is for a person of 100, 150, 200 and 300 pounds. Your weight will probably fall between the columns, requiring you to *guestimate* your approximate Caloric expenditure. Depending on how vigorous the exercise you can add or subtract between 10 and 20 calories for every ten pounds you weigh over or under the columns surrounding your actual weight. This is one place us heavy weights get a break; we actually burn more Calories than skinny folks do!

Exercise is extremely important to arthritic as well as cardiac patients. When my father had his first heart attack or coronary occlusion over forty years ago, he was told to

ACTIVITY	100 LBS	150 LBS	200 LBS	300 LBS
Aerobic dancing (low impact)	115	172	230	345
Aerobics step training, 4" step (beginner)	145	218	290	435
Aerobics, slide training (basic)	150	225	300	435
Backpacking with 10 lb. load	180	270	360	540
Backpacking with 20 lb. load	200	300	400	600
Backpacking with 30 lb. load	235	352	470	705
Badminton	150	225	300	450
Basketball (game)	220	330	440	660
Basketball (leisurely, nongame)	130	195	260	390
Bicycling, 10 mph (6 minutes/mile)	125	188	250	375
Bicycling, 13 mph (4.6 minutes/mile)	200	300	400	600
Billiards	45	68	90	135
Bowling	55	82	110	165
Canoeing, 2.5 mph	70	105	140	210
Canoeing, 4.0 mph	135	202	270	405
Croquet	60	90	120	180
Cross country snow skiing, intense	330	495	660	990
Cross country snow skiing, leisurely	155	232	310	465
Cross country snow skiing, moderate	220	330	440	660
Dancing (noncontact)	100	150	200	300
Dancing (slow)	55	82	110	165
Gardening, moderate	90	135	180	270
Golfing (walking, w/o cart)	100	150	200	300
Golfing (with a cart)	70	105	140	210

Handball	230	345	460	690
Hiking with a 10 lb. load	180	270	360	540
Hiking with a 20 lb. load	200	300	400	600
Hiking with a 30 lb. load	235	352	470	705
Hiking, no load	155	232	310	465
Housework	90	135	180	270
Ironing	50	75	100	150
Jogging, 5 mph (12 minutes/mile)	185	278	370	555
Jogging, 6 mph (10 minutes/mile)	230	345	460	690
Mopping	85	128	170	255
Mowing	135	202	270	405
Ping Pong	90	135	180	270
Raking	75	112	150	225
Raquetball	205	308	410	615
Rowing (leisurely)	75	112	150	225
Rowing machine	180	270	360	540
Running, 08 mph (7.5 minutes/mile)	305	458	610	915
Running, 09 mph (6.7 minutes/mile)	330	495	660	990
Running, 10 mph (6 minutes/mile)	350	525	700	1050
Scrubbing the floor	140	210	280	420
Scuba diving	190	285	380	570
Shopping for groceries	60	90	120	180
Skipping rope	285	428	570	855
Snow shoveling	195	292	390	585
Snow skiing, downhill	130	195	260	390

Soccer	195	292	390	585
Squash	205	308	410	615
Stair climber machine	160	240	320	480
Stair climbing	140	210	280	420
Swimming (25 yards/minute)	120	180	240	360
Swimming (50 yards/minute)	225	338	450	675
Table Tennis	90	135	180	270
Tennis	160	240	320	480
Tennis (doubles)	110	165	220	330
Trimming hedges	105	158	210	315
Vacuuming	75	112	150	225
Volleyball (game)	120	180	240	360
Volleyball (leisurely)	70	105	140	210
Walking, 2 mph (30 minutes/mile)	60	90	120	180
Walking, 3 mph (20 minutes/mile)	80	120	160	240
Walking, 4 mph (15 minutes/mile)	100	150	200	300
Washing the car	75	112	150	225
Waterskiing	160	240	320	480
Waxing the car	100	150	200	300
Weeding	100	150	200	300
Weight training (40 sec. between sets)	255	382	510	765
Weight training (60 sec. between sets)	190	285	380	570
Weight training (90 sec. between sets)	125	188	250	375
Window cleaning	75	112	150	225

reduce his activity drastically. He had to move his bedroom from the second to the first floor to avoid steps. He was told to stay at bed rest for weeks, both in the hospital and after he got home a month and a half after his myocardial infarction. When he was allowed to resume activity, he was warned not to exert himself ... ever! That was how heart disease was treated in those days. When I went to medical school a decade later, they were still advocating inactivity for heart patients. Sad to say, we were not curing heart disease, we were creating *cardiac cripples*.

Today we know better. The heart is a muscle. In addition, like any muscle of the body it improves and strengthens with *prudent* exercise. Most important, the increased circulation of blood provides increased oxygen to nourish its hungering muscle cells. Think about this; in most cases, it is a sedentary lifestyle that causes heart disease. It is thus unlikely that a sedentary lifestyle will improve your cardiac status. **Check with your cardiologist!**

Prudent exercise, on the other hand, can prevent heart disease ... and it will in most cases improve dramatically an already diseased or damaged heart. It does the same for arthritis as far as prevention and improvement are concerned.

So what do we mean by, *"Prudent exercise?"* First of all, it must be designed for *you* specifically! This means supervision and approval of your physician; careful adherence to the prescribed program by you, and consideration of all points covered in the following pages. It is strongly recommended that you take this book with you when you discuss your exercise and fitness program with your medical advisor so there will be no misunderstanding of what is intended by either of you.

Talk to your physician about working out in arthritis rehab program to get you started in the right direction and to create a program fir you.

The exercise you need to improve your joints is best if it can also be an *aerobic* program. An aerobic exercise is one that causes you to breathe deeply and increase your pulse rate to *your ideal exercise pulse rate for a prolonged time* ... eventually 45 minutes to one hour per day. The purpose of an aerobic exercise program is to build cardiovascular and cardiopulmonary strength and endurance; in other words, to strengthen your heart, lungs and circulatory system so they will function most efficiently and have adequate reserve in distressful and emergency situations while improving your joints

More about Aerobics for People with Limited Mobility

Fortunately, there are numerous practical options some of which we have mentioned; let us look in some more detail.

Swimming and pool exercise

For a person with limited mobility water exercises may prove ideal for several reasons, because it presents a range of resistance to the muscles with markedly reduced weight bearing. In some cases, you can even use a walker or special wheelchair in the exercise pool. There are counter current pools available for installation in private residences or apartment and condominium facilities where you adjust the water current flow so you can swim in place or walk with a specific measured challenge.

Water walking can be an excellent option for people with weight bearing problems or arthritic hip, knee or ankle joints. By using a pool noodle, a buoyant foam tube, under your arms or buttock while in the water, you can actually float in one place while moving your legs as though walking, thus getting considerable aerobic benefits. A person who cannot swim nor has mobility handicaps must exercise in water with caution and never go in a pool unsupervised. You might also consider wearing a life jacket or an AquaJogger, a buoyant strap on belt to make you safer in the water. In most areas, water aerobic classes are readily available.

If you can swim at all, try working up to swimming 30 minutes to an hour a day or at least three times a week. Think you can't do that? Most people are limited to short distances swimming by their ability to coordinate their breathing. If that's your problem, try swimming with a snorkel. That will let you breath without having to bring your head out of the water and you will find you can swim what seems almost indefinitely, but for sure 30 to 60 minutes. Swimming is an excellent upper body and endurance builder. Combining swimming with other water exercises burns Calories at a high rate and is very aerobic.

Bicycles stationary or mobile

Stationary bicycles are readily available to the mobility-challenged person who retains the ability to move his or her legs. They come in two main styles, the most common configured like a normal bike or a recumbent style, which is more comfortable for someone who as difficulty sitting in a saddle type seat. If one is able to ride a regular bike but has difficulty bearing weight for prolonged periods, a standard bike may work quite well.

Arm only aerobics for those with upper body ability

only

Even if you have absolutely no use of your legs, aerobic exercise is still within your reach. An *arm ergometer*, a device that looks almost like an inverted stationary bicycle, is available in clubs or for home use. The user sits facing peddles, but grasps them with his or her hands rather than peddling with the feet. They rotate exactly like a bicycle but are powered by your arms providing excellent aerobic exercise.

In addition, there are numerous seated circulation workouts, seated weight workouts and some leg strengthening exercises that might require standing but not walking. Exercise leaders are available on DVD or easily followed programs on TV. Of course, for people still able to walk even just a few steps, it is possible to get a significant workout using walkers or wheelchairs as mentioned before. If you are easily tired out, concentrate on short exercise intervals and repeat several times a day building up your endurance.

In all cases, it is important that if you are of limited mobility always discuss your exercise plans with your health-care professional.

If you think you are unable to exercise, consider my mother in law who had open-heart surgery to replace a defective heart valve when she was 83 years old. In addition, she had a cardiac pacemaker installed. For at least a decade before her surgery, she had not walked more than 100 feet at a time without sitting down for a prolonged rest. Within two days of her surgery, we started her on her walking program. It started with a walk from her bed to the bathroom less than ten feet away. The next day we walked her out into the hall a few feet, to a chair, and then back to her bed. She did that four times that day and it exhausted her. The next day we walked her in the hospital hall for about 50 feet, back to the chair and after a brief rest another 50-foot walk, and back to bed. We did that routine about six times that day. The next day she did about 100 feet of hallway about ten different times. She was surprised to discover that was about a fifth of a mile.

Her walks increased daily and by the time she left the hospital ten days post surgery, she was doing about a mile a day in the halls of the hospital in divided doses. She left the hospital about five days earlier than her surgeon expected her to and he credited her rapid recovery on her daily forced walks.

When we got her home, she started walking outside or in shopping centers when the weather was too inclement. Within four weeks of her hospital discharge, she was walking an hour non-stop and clipping off three miles, or a mile every twenty minutes. That's a very comfortable and easy pace for most people. Today she walks a mile in 16 to 17 minutes with surprising ease for a 90 year old. She walks four miles a day six or seven days a week with a proud bounce to her stride and is healthier and more active than she has been in the past thirty years. *In addition, when the weather is good ... she plays nine holes of golf a week "with the girls!"*

Set your goals in her footsteps!

Discuss your walking plans with your personal medical advisor. Show him or her this book and decide at what level you should begin ... and then begin ... today! If it's from your bed to the toilet and back, so be it. If you can walk a few hundred feet in the hall, so be it. If you can walk a mile, however slow, great! So be it! Wherever you can start ... start ... but start today! And if it goes well today, then go a bit further tomorrow, and a bit further each succeeding day until you can walk an hour. And when you can walk an hour a day, pick up the speed a little each day, which will lengthen the distance of your one-hour walk each day. And continue picking up the speed of your walk until you reach *your ideal exercise pulse rate*. Then as your general health and cardiac and pulmonary fitness improve, you will be able to walk faster and further in that hour while maintaining your ideal exercise pulse rate; **for now do what you can do comfortably!**

CHAPTER 17

JOINT REPLACEMENT

You use at least one joint with every move you make, so when a joint problem like inflammation and arthritis develops you will feel it immediately as pain and stiffness. When the cartilage lining a joint surface becomes rough, dried, infected, inflamed or worn, the bony surfaces of the joint begin rubbing against each other, causing pain. When this occurs first efforts at treatment should be conservative and aimed at reduction of pain, maintenance of function and prevention of permanent damage.

When all other available treatments have failed, the last resort option might be considered which is surgical joint repair or replacement.

The most common joint replacement operations are knee and/or hip replacement. These procedures both provide a safe, reliable means of easing your pain and helping you return to an active and most often normal and pain free life.

Knee Replacement Surgery

Total knee replacement surgery removes a diseased or damaged knee joint and replaced it with an artificial joint called a prosthesis. There are several types of knee prostheses available today and new developments are continually being researched and engineered. These developments include both design and materials.

During replacement surgery, one, two or all three of the knee's parts will be replaced. Once the damaged parts of the knee joint are replaced with smoothly working parts the joint will again function much similarly to a natural knee and will ease the pain experienced before surgery. Function should be restored to permit a more normal lifestyle.

Hip Replacement Surgery

A hip prosthesis should provide a smooth-working joint as would a healthy hip, but is made of metal and plastic or ceramic materials. The hip joint is a ball-and-socket joint that allows your leg to move at several angles and directions. It must be strong enough to bear your body weight above the hips. The ball portion of the joint, at the top of the thighbone, fits into the socket at the pelvis allowing the ball to move easily and painlessly in the socket. During the hip replacement surgery, the ball-and-socket joint is removed. A new metal cup-like socket lined with plastic is inserted in the pelvis to replace the rough bone of your own socket. A metal ball and stem will replace the rough bone and cartilage at the top of your thighbone. After a recovery period of a few weeks to months, you should be able to move easily and painlessly, with few limitations in movement.

Having had both of my hips replaced two years apart I can vouch for the fact that the day after each surgery I had less pain than I'd felt for the month before surgery. I was able to walk comfortably within days and felt fully recovered with in three months. I have to admit I'm glad I don't have three hips, but I'd never put off this surgery if I had any real untreatable discomfort reduced function in any joint. The fact is that diseased joint replacement with artificial ones has been a successful form of treatment for more than 30 years and has helped thousands-crippled by arthritis, injury, and disease-to function normally without pain.

Hand and wrist joint replacement
Joint closest to the fingertip

These joints are not a good candidate for joint replacement, as the bones are very small and do not hold the implants well. The best treatment for advanced arthritis at these joints is fusion and function is only minimally compromised by the lack of motion while pain is relieved.

Joint second joints from the fingertip

Hand function, especially grasping would be severely hindered by fusion of this joint so replacement is recommended here. There have been numerous prosthetic joints designed for this joint replacement, but only the silicone inter-positional arthroplasty has stood the test of time. These joints are made of silicone rubber and have a flexible hinge in the middle and stems at the ends that insert into the shaft of the bone.

Joint third joint from the fingertip

Silicone joint replacement of this joint has produced excellent long-term results.

Thumb-wrist basal joint

This joint is exposed to very high stresses with normal activities, so arthritis of this joint is very common, especially in women. The most common joint replacement procedure for the thumb base is done with natural material. This procedure uses the patient's own tendon to stabilize the thumb. The patient's own tendon is curled to form the new joint cushion and to resurface the joint, providing stability and pain relief. Long-term results have been excellent.

Wrist joint

Wrist arthritis is best treated with surgical joint cleaning or fusion rather than joint replacement. Most wrist-joint prostheses today are investigational and rather unstable and are usually used in extremely low activity patients with painful osteoarthritis or rheumatoid arthritis.

Shoulder joint replacement

The shoulder is perhaps the most complicated joint in the body and if non-operative treatments fail, shoulder replacement surgery may be needed. There a number of different types of shoulder replacements available today. The usual total shoulder replacement involves replacing the arthritic joint surfaces with a highly polished metal ball attached to a stem, and a plastic socket. Patients who have bone-on-bone osteoarthritis with intact rotator cuff tendons are probably good candidates for conventional total shoulder replacement. Another type of shoulder replacement is called reverse total shoulder replacement and is used for people who have completely torn rotator cuffs or have had a previous shoulder replacement that failed.

Spine replacement and fusion surgery

Neurosurgeons and orthopedic surgeons have engaged in surgical research in hopes of being able to offer an alternative to lumbar spinal fusion surgery. This research has led to the promising development of artificial spinal discs.

The spine is a spring like column made of up bones and discs. The blocks of bone, called vertebrae, provide the support and structure of the spine. The spinal discs are in between the bones and act like a shock absorber between the vertebrae. These discs also contribute to the flexibility and motion of the spinal column. As a normal part of aging, the water content of the discs gradually diminishes which can cause the disc to flatten out and even develop tears or cracks. These degenerative discs may cause severe debilitating pain with movement. For years, spinal fusion has been the major treatment for back pain. The purpose and advantage of artificial disc replacement over spinal fusion is to replace the worn out disc, while preserving the motion at the deteriorated spinal level. Artificial disc replacement is still considered experimental and most of the research has been carried out in Europe. To avoid complications that could arise from artificial disc replacement surgery, careful selection of patients by the surgeon is critical. The best candidates for spinal disc replacement are adults with only one symptomatic degenerative disc. In addition, patients whose bone may be weak or osteoporotic due to aging, or other bone disorder, may develop problems if the implant settles into the weak bone. Current research indicates, the clinical diagnoses most fitting for artificial disc replacement include symptomatic degenerative disc disease and post-discectomy syndrome which is persistent back pain following previous surgery to remove a herniated disc.

Ankle replacement

Ankle replacement is too aimed at resurfacing damaged ankle joints with mechanical parts that allow continued ankle motion and function without pain. The other option is fusion, which diminished some function but will eliminate pain. Like hip and knee replacement parts, ankle prostheses are constructed of metal and plastic and may, with time wear out. Patients who are best served by ankle replacement are those who will put low mechanical demands on their artificial joints, usually these are lightweight patients who need to stand and walk with limited or no pain.

Elbow joint replacement

Elbow joint replacement can effectively treat pain caused by arthritis of the elbow. The procedure is also becoming used in aging adults to replace joints damaged by fractures. The artificial elbow is considered successful by more than 90% of replacement patients. The most common reason for an artificial elbow replacement is still arthritis.

There is a great amount of continuing research going on in the field of joint replacement and new surgical methods, prostheses and materials are constantly being developed. The future for this type treatment is bright, but it must be remembered that surgical joint replacement should be help off until all other treatment forms have been exhausted.

CHAPTER 18

ALTERNATIVE MEDICINE

It is important to have been diagnosed with whatever form of arthritis you may have by a health care provider who has conventional medical training and experience with arthritis patients. Proven conventional treatments for arthritic diseases should never be replaced with alternative treatments that are unproven.

Always tell your health care providers about any supplements or medications, either prescription or over-the-counter products you are using or considering.

Prescribed medicines may have to be adjusted if you are also using alternative therapy. Supplements may often interact with other medications affecting how the body responds to them. Pharmacists can also be a helpful source of information about dietary supplements; it is wise to get all medications and supplements form one pharmacist who thus knows of everything you are taking.

It is most important to know whether or not scientific research has proven that a therapy works and its claims are true and what its mechanisms of action really are. Women who may be pregnant or are nursing, or parents who are thinking of using alternative medication to treat a child, should use extra caution and be sure to consult their pediatrician.

Botanicals and other dietary supplements

There is not a great amount of long term and rigorous research available on the effectiveness and safety of botanical and food supplements that people ingest in hopes of treating their arthritis. Supplements made from plants and used for medicinal purposes, referred to as herbal medicines, can have effects as powerful as those of drugs can. Many conventional drugs, in fact, originally came from plants. Thus, it is very important to be as informed as possible about the safety of any supplement you may be using.

Special Diets

It is probable that certain foods affect the progress of some arthritic diseases. Some foods that possibly worsen the symptoms of arthritis are the nightshade family of plants that include white potatoes, tomatoes, eggplants, and peppers. Also dairy products, citrus fruits, acidic foods, sweets, coffee, and animal protein may cause certain arthritic conditions to progress and worsen.

How our digestive systems handle foods we eat affects the immune system. Many of the arthritic diseases appear related to aberrant immune system functions, so a connection between diet and the disease most likely exists. Certain fats from animal sources, as well as from corn and sunflower oils, break down into substances that can cause inflammation once in the body.

Acupuncture

Acupuncture developed as a part of traditional Chinese medicine. Many arthritis patients have tried acupuncture to treat their arthritis pain. There have been many good research studies showing acupuncture to help relieve pain associated with arthritis. Acupuncture has minimal side effects, if any and few complications from acupuncture have been reported to the FDA. It is most important to find a licensed and certified practitioner.

Magnets

Magnets produce a type of energy called magnetic fields. Products that contain magnets intended to help treat arthritic symptoms include shoe insoles, clothing, wraps for parts of the body, and mattress pads.

Research to date does not support claims that magnets are effective for treating pain of any source.

Pregnant women or patients using pacemakers, defibrillators, or insulin pumps, or medication patches should not use magnets. Magnets continue to be studied because there have been some early vague findings indicating possible benefits for pain, physical function, and stiffness.

Hydrotherapy

Hydrotherapy or balneotherapy is the use of water for therapeutic purposes, such as bathing in heated water, as from hot springs or the sea; mineral baths; and water-jet massages. Hydrotherapy is used in traditional Western medicine as well as in alternative treatments, including whirlpool baths for athletic injuries and ice for sprains.

While the above mentioned hydrotherapy modes may be found helpful to arthritis patients, internal treatments using water, such as colon irrigation or drinking specially treated water have not been proven effective in the treatment of arthritis.

Most important when entering into a treatment program including alternative medicine practices, is that you confer with your physician to get his or her opinion of the procedures, their possible interaction with your traditional medications and treatments, any possible dangers and to make him or her aware of all procedures or supplements you might be adding to your treatments.

CHAPTER 19

FUTURE OUTLOOK

Recently approved drugs and continuing research into new medications, surgical procedures and prosthetic designs and materials offer patients continues hope and new options. As the population ages arthritis will become an ever-growing problem there will surely be increased research and development into new and improved treatments. Much of this research and development will be toward a better understanding of our immune system and control of its malfunctions. This in mind, the future for arthritis patients is brighter than ever before for both prevention and treatment of the many arthritic diseases.

APPENDIX I

ARTHRITIS RELATED STATISTICS

PREVALENCE OF ARTHRITIS

An estimated 46 million adults in the United States reported being told by a doctor that they have some form of arthritis, rheumatoid arthritis, gout, lupus, or fibromyalgia. One in five (over 21%) adults in the United States report having doctor diagnosed arthritis. In 2003–2005, 50% of adults 65 years and over reported an arthritis diagnosis. By 2030, an estimated 67 million of Americans aged 18 years or older are projected to have doctor-diagnosed arthritis. An estimated 294,000 children under age 18 have some form of arthritis or rheumatic condition; this represents approximately one in every 250 children.

Prevalence of Specific Types of Arthritis
The most common form of arthritis is osteoarthritis. Other common rheumatic conditions include gout, fibromyalgia and rheumatoid arthritis. An estimated 21 million adults have osteoarthritis. An estimated 2.1 million

adults are affected by rheumatoid arthritis. An estimated 5.1 million adults report having a doctor diagnosis of gout. An estimated 3.7 million adults have fibromyalgia.

Prevalence of Arthritis by Age/Race/Gender

Of persons aged 18–44, 7.9% (8.7 million) report doctor-diagnosed arthritis. Of persons aged 45–64, 29.3% (20.5 million) report doctor-diagnosed arthritis. Of persons aged 65+, 50.0% (17.2 million) report doctor-diagnosed arthritis, 28.3 million women and 18.1 million men report doctor-diagnosed arthritis, 3.1 million Hispanic adults report doctor-diagnosed arthritis, 4.6 million Non-Hispanic Blacks report doctor-diagnosed arthritis. An estimated 294,000 children under age 18 have some form of arthritis or rheumatic condition; this represents approximately one in every 250 children.

Overweight/Obesity and Arthritis (adult aged 18)

People who are overweight or obese report more doctor-diagnosed arthritis than thinner people, 16% of under/normal weight adults report doctor-diagnosed arthritis, 21.7% of overweight and 30.6% among obese Americans report doctor-diagnosed arthritis, 66% of adults with doctor-diagnosed arthritis, are overweight or obese (compared with 53% of adults without doctor-diagnosed arthritis). Weight loss of as little as 11 pounds reduces the risk of developing knee osteoarthritis among women by 50%.

Physical Activity and Arthritis

Almost 44% of adults with doctor-diagnosed arthritis report no leisure time physical activity compared with 36% of adults without arthritis. Among older adults with knee osteoarthritis, engaging in moderate physical activity at least 3 times per week can reduce the risk of arthritis-related disability by 47%.

Disability/Limitations and Arthritis

State-specific prevalence estimates of arthritis-attributable work limitation show a high impact of arthritis on working-age (18-64 years) adults in all U.S. states, ranging from a low of 3.4% to a high of 15% of adults with arthritis in this age group. Approximately 5% of ALL U.S. adults between the ages of 18 and 64 in this age group are affected by arthritis-attributable work limitation. Approximately 1 in 3 people with arthritis in this age group report arthritis-attributable work limitation Arthritis and other rheumatic conditions are a leading cause of disability in the United States. Among all civilian, non-institutionalized U.S. adults 8.8% (19 million) report both doctor-diagnosed and arthritis attributable "activity limitations." Nearly 41% of adults with doctor-diagnosed arthritis report arthritis-attributable activity limitations. Among adults with doctor-diagnosed arthritis, many report significant limitations in vital activities such as:

❖ walking 1/4 mile—6 million
❖ stooping/bending/kneeling—7.8 million
❖ climbing stairs—4.8 million
❖ social activities such as church and family gatherings—2.1 million

Among all civilian, non-institutionalized U.S. adults, aged 18-64, 4.8% (8.2 million) report both doctor diagnosed arthritis and arthritis-attributable work limitations, 30.6% of adults aged 18-64 with doctor-diagnosed arthritis report an arthritis-attributable work limitation.

Health Related Quality of Life (HRQOL) and Arthritis

Persons with doctor-diagnosed arthritis have significantly worse HRQOL than those without arthritis. People with doctor-diagnosed report more than twice as many unhealthy days and three times as many days with activity limitations in the past month than those without arthritis.

Arthritis Healthcare Utilization
Hospitalizations

In 1997, there were an estimated 744,000 hospitalizations with a principal diagnosis of arthritis (3% of all hospitalizations).

Outpatient Care

There were 36.5 million ambulatory care visits for arthritis and other rheumatic conditions in 1997, or nearly 4% of all ambulatory care visits that year.

Arthritis-Related Mortality

From 1979-1998, the annual number of arthritis and other related rheumatic conditions (AORC) deaths rose from 5,537 to 9,367. Three categories of AORC account for almost 80% of deaths: diffuse connective tissue diseases (34%), other specified rheumatic conditions (23%), and rheumatoid arthritis (22%). In 1979, the crude death rate from AORC was 2.46 per 100,000 populations. In 1998, it was 3.48 per 100,000 population; rates age-standardized to the year 2000 population were 2.75 and

3.51, respectively.

Arthritis Costs

In 2003, the total cost attributed to arthritis and other rheumatic conditions in the United States was 128 billion dollars, up from 86.2 billion dollars in 1997. Medical expenditures (direct costs) for arthritis and other rheumatic conditions in 2003 were 80.8 billion dollars, up from 51.1 billion in 1997. Earnings losses (indirect costs) for arthritis and other rheumatic conditions in 2003 were 47 billion dollars, up from 35.1 billion in 1997.

Mental/Emotional Health and Arthritis

Arthritis is strongly associated with major depression (attributable risk of 18.1%), probably through its role in creating functional limitation.

Total Joint Replacements in Arthritis

In 2003, there were 418,000 total knee replacements performed, primarily for arthritis.

APPENDIX II
QUIT SMOKING NOW

Dr. Seiden believes in prevention being more important than the cure, therefore, the detrimental side effects of smoking are well documented and many times, smoking increases Arthritis symptoms and suffering.

Dr. Seiden has written and published a full course on how to Quit Smoking Now and he gives this away to anyone who has a desire to quit or simply wants some more information.

Please visit BoomerBookSeries.com/QuitSmokingNow.php and download your free 66 page e-book to Quit Smoking Now!

RECOMMENDED READING

THE ARTHRITIS HELPBOOK BY KATE LORIG & JAMES FRIES
ISBN: 0738210706

THE ANTI-INFLAMMATION DIET AND RECIPE BOOK, PROTECT YOURSELF AND YOUR FAMILY FROM HEART DISEASE, ARTHRITIS, DIABETES, ALLERGIES AND MORE BY N.D. JESSICA K. BLACK
ISBN: 0897934857

THE CLEVELAND CLINIC GUIDE TO ARTHRITIS BY MD JOHN D. CLOUGH
ISBN: 1427799563

LIVING WELL WITH CHRONIC PAIN BY JUDE WILLHOFF
ISBN: 1-932344-84-5 - BOOMER BOOK SERIES

ARTHRITIS: THE CURE - THE LAST BOOK YOU'LL EVER NEED ON ARTHRITIS BY MD GEORGE TILDEN
ISBN: 1441465766

About The Author(s)

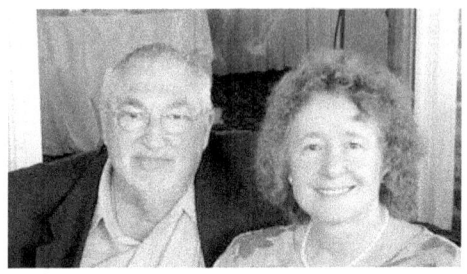

Othniel J. Seiden, M.D.
Jane L. Bilett, Ph.D.

The human animal is intended to be active throughout life and Arthritis, in its many forms has become the *number one debilitating disease* interfering with our mobility and continued function.

Jane L. Bilett, PhD has practiced Clinical Psychology for over 30 years and Othniel J. Seiden, MD medicine for well over 40 years. In addition, Othniel has experienced the disease from the patient's point of view having had two hip replacements.

Together, Jane and Othniel have helped hundreds of individuals to cope with these handicapping diseases. To achieve the best possible mobility and active life through the senior years requires both prevention and cure of these diseases. With their cumulative experience dealing with the psychological and medical aspects of arthritis, they are most qualified to help you retain the best life quality you can hope for!

More From Othniel

Health

5 HTP The Serotonin Connection:
*The Natural Supplement that helps
you be in control of your mind and body!*
ISBN: 1519148445
5-HTP and Depression Management:
Available in Kindle Only
5HTP and Memory Loss Management with:
Available in Kindle Only
5 HTP PMS and Menopause:
Available in Kindle Only
Coping with Arthritis:
ISBN: 151941353X
Coping with BPH:
*Benign Prostatic Hypertrophy
Male, over 45, you probably have it!*
Available in Kindle Only
Coping with Colorectal Cancer:
*Prevention and Cure of theSecond Leading
Cause of Cancer Deaths*
Available in Kindle Only
Coping with Fibromyalgia:
It's not in your head, it's a disease!
ISBN: 1519438311

Coping with Prostate Cancer:
> *Prevention and Cure*
> *of Man's Most Common Cancer*
> **ISBN: 1519438737**

Heart of a Woman:
> *Prevetion and Cure of the #1 Killer in Women*
> **ISBN: 1519441533**

Heavy and Healthy:
> *Forget Your Weight and Get Fit!*
> **ISBN: 1519495412**

Quit Smoking Now!:
> *The Program to Help You*
> *Quit Smoking Now and Forever!*
> **ISBN: 1519495781**

Sharpening the Aging Mind:
> *Methods, Tricks & Tips to*
> *Keep Your Mind Super Sharp*
> **ISBN: 1519496028**

Sleep Disorders Management:
> **Available in Kindle Only**

The Second half begins at 50:
> *Your Longevity Handbook*
> **ISBN: 1519496389**

Walk!:
> *Walk Your Way to Great Health & Long Life*
> **Available in Kindle Only**

Weight & Appetite Management:
> **Available in Kindle Only**

Relationships:

Adultery Case Histories:
Why People Cheat on Their Partners
Available in Kindle Only
Communing with the Dead:
Death Needn't Part You
ISBN: 1519190085
Foreplay:
The True Focus of Great Sex
ISBN: 1519440979
Sex in the Golden Years:
The Best Sex Ever, Stay Sexually Active for Life
ISBN: 1519495927
The Big O:
Male & Female Multiple Orgasms
ISBN: 1519496109
The Hospice Experience:
Making Your Most Important Final Decision
ISBN: 1519496281
When Your Spouse Dies:
A widow's & widower's handbook
ISBN: 151949646X

Jewish Fiction

Padre Pio:
*The Capuchin – the life of Padre Pio -
St. Pio of Pietrelcina
Sex, Horror & Violence vs. Unyielding Faith!*
ISBN: 1519495684

Seed of Avraham:
A 4000 Year History of the Jewish Family...
ISBN: 1519495811

Shtetl:
The Story of a Life No More...
As told from the hereafter
ISBN: 1519496036

The Cartographer:
1492
ISBN: 151949615X

The Condemned Voyage:
The S.S. St. Louis - 1939
Available in Kindle Only

The Crusades:
The Jewish World of the 12th Century
Available in Kindle Only

The Death of Berlin:
A Story of Hollocaust Survival and Revenge
Available in Kindle Only

The Remnant:
The Jewish Resistance in WWII
ISBN: 1519496346

The Uprising of Babi Yar:
The Syrets Deathcamp
Available in Kindle Only

Miscellaneous

Guaranteed Routes to Success for Writers:
A Road Map Through Today's
Dramatic Changes in Publishing
Available in Kindle Only

Joy of Volunteering:
Working and Surviving in Developing Countries
ISBN: 1519495587

So You Want to Write a Book:
ISBN: 1519496079

PLEASE LEAVE A REVIEW FOR

COPING WITH ARTHRITIS

ON AMAZON.COM

ALSO AVAILABLE IN KINDLE!

www.ingramcontent.com/pod-product-compliance
Lightning Source LLC
Chambersburg PA
CBHW071405280526
45787CB00001B/448